Enhancing the Lives of Adults with Disabilities

An Orientation Manual

Third Edition

Dale DiLeo

Training Resource Network, Inc. • St. Augustine, Florida, USA

Third Edition, 2000

This publication is sold with the understanding that the publisher is not engaged in rendering legal, financial, medical, or other such services. If legal advice or other such expert assistance is required, a competent professional in the appropriate field should be sought. All brand and product names are trademarks or registered trademarks of their respective companies.

Printed in the United States of America

Published by Training Resource Network, Inc., PO Box 439, St. Augustine, FL 32085-0439, USA

We invite you to visit our web site at www.trninc.com or e-mail us at info@trninc.com. You also can order tollfree at 866-823-9800.

Library of Congress Cataloging in Publication Data
DiLeo, Dale, date.
   Enhancing the lives of adults with disabilities : an orientation manual / Dale DiLeo.--
3rd ed.
      p. cm.
   Includes biographical references and index.
   ISBN-13 978-1-83302-38-2
    1. Developmentally disabled--Services for--United States. 2. Developmentally disabled--Rehabilitation--United States. 3. Handicapped--Services for--United States. 4. Handicapped--Rehabilitation--United States. I. Title

HV1570.5.U6 D55 2000
362.1'968--dc21   00-062988

Contents

Acknowledgments

The material presented in *Enhancing the Lives of Adults with Disabilities* reflects a view of how services for people with disabilities best can be provided. I have had the gift of being influenced in developing this outlook by forward-thinking professionals who challenged the status quo: Mark Gold, Lou Brown, Burton Blatt, Gunnar Dybwad, Tom Bellamy, John O'Brien, Herb Lovett, Wolf Wolfensberger, and many others. I hope the information provided does justice to their work.

The concepts presented here also represent an evolution in the field that parallels my own career. My twenty-five-year journey providing services to people with disabilities started with time spent delivering services in the only types of facilities that existed at the time: institutions, group homes, day habilitation programs, and sheltered workshops. More recently, I have worked in partnership with people in their quest for real jobs, true friendships, and homes of their own. As my own work changed, I watched as people with disabilities succeeded in their communities. One person at a time, each taught me about new approaches, at the same time challenging my beliefs about how services should be and what they should look like.

This manual originally was funded and developed by the New Hampshire Division of Mental Health and Developmental Services (NHDMHDS) and the Institute on Disability at the University of New Hampshire, and further developed in Massachusetts through the state's Department of Mental Retardation (DMR). I would like to give special thanks to Mike Shields, training director of NHDMHDS and Jan Nisbet, director of the Institute for their guidance, and to Sam O'Brien for his dedication to orientation training in Massachusetts. I also would like to thank the following individuals and their affiliated agencies for their comments and contributions to the original text:

Cassin, C.	Massachusetts Department of Mental Retardation
Colby, W.	New England College
Dubois, G.	Laconia Developmental Services
Fryer, C.	Easter Seals, New Hampshire
Gersterberger, R.	Region 12 Developmental Services
Hoeveler, F.K.	Concord, New Hampshire Parent Information Program
Langle, S.	NHDMHDS
Langton, D.	DL Networks
Lepore, R.	NHDMHDS
Myatt, C.	Lakes Region Community Services Council
Paine, A.	NHDMHDS
Parlor, K.	Region VI Area Agency for Developmental Services
Platts, B.	Northern NH Mental Health & Developmental Services
Prince, H.	Center of Hope
Robichaud, A.	NHDMHDS
Treisner, D.	Institute on Disability, University of New Hampshire
Tuller, J.	Massachusetts Department of Mental Retardation
Urban, L.	Greater Nashua Child Care
Woodfin, D.	New Hampshire Disability Rights Center

Enhance

verb (in. hans') to make higher or greater as in reputation, beauty, quality, etc.
— *Funk and Wagnalls Standard Dictionary*

About the Author

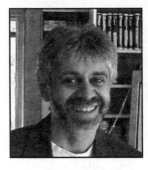

Dale DiLeo has been an advocate for people with disabilities for twenty-five years. He directs Training Resource Network, Inc., an international publishing and consultation firm located in St. Augustine, Florida. He has authored numerous books and is the publisher of the popular employment newsletter, *Supported Employment InfoLines*. Dale has provided training throughout the US, Canada, and Europe on community inclusion for persons with disabilities. He has consulted with many state and private agencies, public schools, universities, professional associations, and corporations. He is the past-president of the board of the Association for Persons in Supported Employment. He has presented keynotes at various international conferences, including the APSE National conference, the European Supported Employment Conference in Oslo, Norway, and the Canadian Conference on Supported Employment in Toronto.

In Memoriam

Over the past few years several leaders of the field, who were also colleagues and friends, passed away. Rebecca McDonald, past president of the Association for Persons in Supported Employment, was a fierce advocate for integration and community employment for people with disabilities. Herb Lovett, author and lecturer, taught us eloquently and humorously about how to respectfully help people with challenging behavior. Dick Lepore, who directed statewide developmental disability services in New Hampshire at the time this manual was first written, later implemented the concept of independent support coordination for people with disabilities in several states. We will miss their voices.

Introduction

You have chosen a career in services for people with disabilities at an exciting time. There has been a dramatic shift in the way people think about services and how they provide support to someone with a disability. The past several years have brought major accomplishments in a number of areas, including new laws, new programs, and new expectations. But most of all, persons with disabilities themselves have accomplished much in their own communities—by living, working, and recreating as our neighbors, co-workers, and friends. Their contributions teach us how we are all more alike than different, and make us realize how much we still need to learn to provide effective services.

> Your role, whether it is in a residence, on a job site, or as a support person in an office, is to enhance opportunities for persons with disabilities to participate in their communities as valued neighbors, productive workers, and good friends.

We have discovered much about service needs by listening better and understanding better what persons with disabilities and their families and friends are saying they want and need. We have learned that services are most successful when individualized needs such as these are met in a community context:

- to be seen, first of all, as an individual
- to have love, friendship, encouragement, and long-lasting relationships
- to be treated as an equal partner with respect and dignity
- to have opportunities to grow and learn skills based not only on need, but on aptitudes and interests
- to have information and experiences to make educated choices and to be heard expressing those choices
- to participate in and contribute to local communities
- to live in a quality home and to work at a satisfying job

Your role, whether it is working with people in their homes, on their job sites, or as a support person in an office, is to work to meet these needs. This will require an understanding of the service system and the resources in your state and your community. Most of all, it will require an understanding of each person with whom you work. Your role is important. Your appearance, dress, attitude, and skills make a difference, and will tell the community a lot about the people you are assisting. **Above all, your personal relationships with the community and the people with whom you work will be critical.**

This orientation manual is designed to assist you in these efforts. Each section provides a brief overview of an introductory subject. It will be important for you to review this material carefully. Ask questions and seek out further information through your supervisor and agency as you become more experienced in your work.

Each section is followed by a brief review session for you to complete. Your trainer or supervisor should go over the information covered with you. I hope you enjoy your work and wish you success.

Part A

An Overview of Disabilities

Labelling People Can Be Harmful

Whenever you read about people with disabilities, you likely will see many terms used to describe their particular disability. Two examples of these you probably have read before are mental illness and developmental disabilities. Terms like these can be useful. People who share something in common are grouped together and this makes it easier to communicate about them.

But these terms are also labels, and labelling a person can be harmful. Focusing on someone's challenges and labelling him or her by them make us forget about the many unique capabilities a person can offer.

> Labels make us think everyone with the label is alike. When a person is called mentally retarded, we have a certain image of him or her. But each individual with mental retardation is a unique person with his or her own dreams, goals, and needs, just like everyone else is.

For example, over the years various labels have been used to classify people labeled with mental retardation, including feebleminded, idiot, imbecile, totally dependent, and custodial. These terms have taken on very negative meanings and images. Like most negative labels, they demean people, unfairly stereotype them, and stress differences rather than abilities. Even neutral words can eventually become words that convey a poor image for a person.

Labels make us forget that each person is an individual. We all hear about the "average person," but have you ever met an "average person?" Each person has unique strengths and needs. When we label a person who has a disability, the label hides capabilities. A person with a disability could be paralyzed and be very intelligent, but a label makes us think only of the paralysis.

Labels tend to make us predict that people will act in certain ways. People tend to act based on the way others expect them to act. When we are responsible to help someone and we think that a person cannot learn to do something, the more likely the person will have trouble accomplishing it. This is because when we reduce our

self-fulfilling prophecy

expectations, we reduce opportunities for positive experiences. This is called a *self-fulfilling prophecy*.

An example of this is when people think someone cannot change—even with learning opportunities. This is not true. All people can do better or worse according to their environment, their attitude, their health, and expectations. Have you ever done something well in one instance and poorly in another? An athlete might run a fast mile during practice. But the fear of failure and the tension of a race might cause him or her to slow down. On the other hand, a musician might have difficulty with a part during practice. But he or she continues to practice with the expectation for success and then plays flawlessly on stage.

> John is a social person who is very curious about his world and the people in it. He could learn to talk, but has been unable to get the communication services he needs. Why?
>
> Because John is labelled pro-foundly retarded. He is blind, has a severe curvature of the spine, and cannot walk or sit up. Program staff always have been taught to do everything for him. He is in a setting with other people labelled as profoundly retarded.
>
> No one expects John to talk. This self-fulfilling prophecy restricts his potential. He is entitled, like all of us, to explore and develop his interests and his capacities as a person with something to contribute.

The self-fulfilling prophecy thus also can work positively for people. The environment and how we feel both influence our abilities to do many things, positively or negatively. When we realistically expect a lot from people, when we believe in their abilities, and when we give them the supports they need, they likely will improve their performance.

Communities Are for Everyone

In recent years, our society has recognized how much the environment affects the abilities of all people, including those with disabilities. A great deal of legislation has been passed to ensure that the environments in which people with disabilities live and work are beneficial.

One result of this is that each year an *individual service plan* should be written for each person. Details on how these plans must be developed and monitored vary from state to state. But certain things are consistent. For instance, a team of people must meet to write this plan. The most important member of the team is the person with a disability. At the meeting, life experiences, goals, and events of the past year are reviewed and put into context. The person's dreams and hopes are explored. New learning experiences and opportunities are determined.

individual service plan

This represents a big change from the past. A plan such as this assumes that all people will learn and grow. It recognizes that people are influenced positively by good environments. This is true not only for people with disabilities, but for all people.

The needs of people go beyond individual plans and beneficial environments. To have a quality life, we all need self-respect as well as the respect of others. We need to feel a part of a community and to have friends, family, and neighbors there.

In spite of recent positive changes, in many places in the US people with disabilities still are segregated and are not provided supports to live and work in their communities. And labels still are commonly used to describe people in their everyday lives.

Unfortunately, it is sometimes easier to view someone as a label rather than as a person who can do some things and not others. It then becomes simple to relegate people to segregated, "safe" environments. It is important to make sure you don't use or create negative self-fulfilling prophecies with the people with whom you work.

People with disabilities are, first and foremost, **people with abilities**. Without assistance, some people cannot take advantage of the opportunities of our society. Without support, the challenges they face may make them vulnerable to abuse or neglect. But just because a person with a disability relies on you for support in some way does not change the fact that he or she is a capable person—someone much more like you than different. After all, who among us has not relied on someone for some sort of support?

Developmental Changes

People change as they grow. Physical growth refers to changes in the body, such as growing taller or gaining weight. Mental growth means changes in thinking and language, including learning to talk, telling the difference between large and small objects, and telling time. These physical and mental changes work together so that individuals grow to do more and more complex things.

Babies crawl, eat with their hands, and are not toilet trained. Children walk and run, eat with utensils, and use the bathroom. At generally predictable times, people begin to demonstrate certain skills. They are examples of behavioral milestones, or changes in the way we act.

Most individuals show similar kinds of physical, mental, and behavioral growth as they age. Each person develops at his or her own speed, but most people develop at similar rates. For example, most babies say their first words between ten and fourteen months. Most children begin to walk by the time they are twelve to eighteen

developmental disability

months old. These are examples of developmental landmarks. A child who does not pass through landmarks at the expected age may have a *developmental disability*.

Functioning, or the ability to successfully negotiate the environment, is a key element in defining a developmental disability. Rather than looking at only causes or labels, focus on the individual's needs, accomplishments, and barriers to community living.

Functional areas are usually grouped in the following way:

1. self-care
2. language
3. learning
4. mobility
5. self-direction
6. independent living
7. economic self-sufficiency

Examples of Developmental Disabilities

The causes and kinds of developmental disabilities are varied. Since you likely will work with many different people, a few examples of developmental disabilities as well as other common disabilities are described in the next pages.

> A developmental disability is based on not achieving certain developmental landmarks in functioning at expected ages.

As you review these terms, remember that a **disability label does not tell us about a person's skills or capabilities.** For example, to best support a person with cerebral palsy, you will need to know the individual well. If the person has provided you with written reports, you may find documents from a physical or occupational therapist or a physician that describe in detail the specific disability. But while reports can provide you with important information, it is knowing the person and his or her family and friends that will be the greatest source to guide you in providing assistance. **It is important to understand the person's goals, hopes, experiences, and capabilities,** as well as his or her particular type of disability.

Cerebral Palsy

Cerebral palsy is a general term. People with cerebral palsy have difficulty controlling some of their body muscles. They may make weak or uncoordinated movements. This is caused by damage to certain areas of the brain. Damage to different parts of the brain causes different forms of cerebral palsy.

Each person with cerebral palsy has very different kinds of abilities and disabilities, and like all of us, **each is a unique individual**. Many people with cerebral palsy have normal or above average intelligence, although sometimes an individual might have other disabilities like blindness, deafness, epilepsy, or mental retardation. People with cerebral palsy may make a number of different kinds of movements. Here are some common examples and the terms used to define them:

Spasticity: involuntary muscle tightening causing resistance to controlled movement

Rigidity: stiffness of the body or limbs

Tremor: shaky muscles when a coordinated movement such as reaching or walking is attempted

Athetosis: slow, uncontrolled, twisting movements

As you can see, these movements are all very different. Most people with cerebral palsy experience a mixture of these.

Spina Bifida

When the spinal cord fails to close, a baby might be born with spina bifida. Like cerebral palsy, these individuals might have a variety of challenges. They might not have a sense of touch or pain in their legs, for example. Or they might have paralysis of their bladder or bowels that prevents them from controlling their bodily functions. Some people need very little assistance while others require intensive support. Once again, you will need to know the capabilities and needs of each person in order to be of help.

Recent medical technology has enabled individuals with a spinal cord disability to participate in many more and varied environments than ever before. As a result, opportunities are becoming more available to **contribute more fully in their communities** as workers, family members, neighbors, and citizens.

Autism

People with autism have difficulty relating to other people. They avoid or may not pay attention to others. They have difficulty communicating. Often, people with autism prefer things to stay the same, becoming upset with small changes in a room or a routine. While individuals with autism all tend to display these behaviors, they vary greatly from person to person.

Autism occurs more often in males than females. Researchers are uncertain of its cause, but believe there is a physical basis. Some individuals may spend hours rocking back and forth, singing to themselves, or moving their hands in front of their eyes. This *self-*

stimulatory behavior, as well as the social and communication difficulties, can interfere with learning more useful and productive ways of behaving.

When a person with autism uses his or her language skills, she or he does not talk to people in usual ways. For example, Barbara sometimes repeats exactly what other people say to her. This is called *echolalia.* Some people may talk only about a single topic, while others hardly speak at all.

Some people with autism have learned how to communicate to others in more effective ways. One promising but still controversial approach being researched is called *facilitated communication.* In this technique, a facilitator may begin by gently assisting the individual to use a keyboard to type out answers to questions. As guidance is faded, the individual learns to type out language more independently. This technique may teach us more about the capabilities of people with autism. Still, since communicating is difficult, it is very important to learn how to understand what the person's patterns of behavior may communicate.

People with autism **should live and work in their communities.** While most of these individuals have some degree of mental retardation, not all do. Some people have unusual and exceptional skills in music, art, movement, memory, and math. Knowing each individual well will help you to better facilitate his or her growth by providing more effective assistance and training.

facilitated communication

> **The following are the federal guidelines for defining a develop-mental disability:**
>
> A disability attributable to mental retardation, cerebral palsy, epilepsy, autism, or a specific learning disability; or any other closely related condition that:
> - originates before age twenty-two
> - has continued or can be expected to continue indefinitely
> - constitutes a severe handicap to the individual's ability to function normally in society.

Mental Retardation

People with mental retardation are individuals who have difficulty learning general knowledge as well as *adaptive behavior.* Adaptive behavior is the way a person adjusts to the environment. When a person has difficulty with adaptive behavior, she or he also will have difficulty meeting expectations for personal independence at his or her age level.

adaptive behavior

There are a number of different definitions of mental retardation. One way of defining it is by an intelligence quotient (IQ). A score of sixty-eight or below on the Stanford-Binet or the Wechsler Intelligence Scale, for example, has been used to indicate a label of mental retardation. By this definition, about 3% of the population would be labelled. A person also must have difficulty functioning in various ways and the difficulty must be present before adulthood.

More recently, professionals have discarded IQ scores in order to define mental retardation differently. The new definition classifies the *needed supports* for each person to function successfully in society.

Another way of looking at mental retardation is to consider how and when the disability began. There are over 200 known causes of mental retardation, and these account for only a quarter of its occurrence. These include genetic disorders such as *Down Syndrome*, infections and intoxications during pregnancy such as rubella, poor environmental factors in early life, or brain damage.

One way of classifying these causes is to group them by genetic problems, pregnancy difficulties, birth difficulties, or problems with the environment after birth. Another way is to classify by medical groupings of causes, including infection, injury, metabolism, and brain disease.

There are a number of recognized classifications that have specific characteristics related to mental retardation. For example, people with *Lesch-Nyhan Syndrome* have great difficulty with motor movement and controlling their behaviors of self-injury. Individuals with *Phenylketonuria (PKU)* often have autistic-like behaviors. People who have *Prader-Willi Syndrome* often are preoccupied with food, usually eating to dangerous excess. *Rett's Syndrome* describes a condition in females who, after normal development, lose previous developmental milestones within the first two years of life, and often display behaviors much like people with autism.

There are a number of other terms that are used to label individuals with mental retardation for purposes of information, funding services, and classification of needs. Again, these labels, while they serve a purpose, also can be harmful. For example, in order to classify levels of functioning, you will see these terms: *borderline, mild, moderate, severe,* and *profound*.

Like any label, these words take on negative stereotypes and self-fulfilling prophecies. While it is necessary to understand the usage of these terms by policy-makers, researchers, and others, it is not in the interests of the individual to use them in referring to him or her.

Although the two are very different, mental retardation is sometimes confused with *mental illness*. Mental retardation, unlike mental illness, is not an illness to be treated. And unlike mental retardation, mental illness can occur

Down Syndrome

> The functional definition of developmental disability is not a label like "autism" or "mental retardation." While understanding these conditions is necessary, it is more important to understand the individual person.

at any age and involves psychological, behavioral, or emotional disturbances with reality.

Even though the two conditions are distinct, people who have developmental disabilities are as susceptible as anyone else to developing mental illness. They should have the same access to community mental health centers for diagnosis, medication, counseling, and crisis support as we all have.

Mental illness and mental retardation are different terms that can be confused with each other. Mental retardation is a lifelong developmental disability related to difficulties with learning. Mental illness can occur at any age and involve disturbances in dealing with life's realities.

Although people with mental retardation typically experience challenges in learning more complex tasks, **it is a mistake to limit anyone's potential.** Like everyone, individuals with retardation are very capable of mastering many complicated functional skills to excel in living, working, and recreating in their communities when given the right support.

Epilepsy

People who have epilepsy have *seizures* caused by changes in the normal, electrical rhythms of the brain. This happens when injured brain cells cannot transmit the correct signal. It's something like an electrical short circuit.

seizures

There are many causes of seizures. These include:
1. head injuries
2. tumors or infections in the brain
3. decrease in oxygen and blood to the brain
4. abnormal development of the brain
5. high fevers (most common in infants and children)
6. chemical imbalances such as low blood sugar

About 7% of the general population have at least one seizure in their lifetime. People who are mentally retarded have a higher incidence. Individuals who have epilepsy **are able to function very capably in the community.** Most people are able to reduce the frequency of seizures with proper medication and health practices.

Specific Learning Disabilities

Individuals with specific learning disabilities have precise difficulties in understanding some aspects of spoken or written language. Because of this, they have difficulty learning and might experience problems in listening, thinking, talking, reading, remembering, writing, or spelling. This results in less than expected achievement.

People with learning disabilities **can learn to compensate and make accommodations to their particular learning style.** With support and training, people with learning disabilities can achieve their fullest capacity.

Other Functional Disabilities

There are a number of other types of disabilities that might cause an individual to have difficulty with day-to-day functioning.

Head Injury

In the fast-paced world in which we live, people receive injuries. When a trauma occurs to the head, a brain injury may result. Depending on the location and extent of the damage, people with head injuries may face a variety of difficulties, including memory loss, confusion, agitation, and problems with walking, coordination, or other uses of the muscles.

People with these types of problems have the added difficulty of dealing with the emotional trauma of a sudden change in skills, sense of self, and other roles related to the injury. As a result, the individual might need support to deal with depression and other related states. Many people with head injuries are able to relearn some of the skills they have lost, and might retain many of the skills they used previously.

Mental Illness

There are many kinds of patterns psychologists recognize to describe people who have various kinds of psychiatric disorders. People may have feelings of deep depression, anxiety, confusion, or even perceptual problems such as hallucinations or delusions. There also may be patterns or cycles in which people predictably go in and out of these experiences.

Since mental illness is a separate kind of disability from developmental disability, some people with developmental disabilities can also have a mental illness. Although rare, this type of challenge has been called having a *dual disability.* Individuals with mental illness, with proper support, counseling, medication, and/or other treatment, can be effective employees and productive citizens.

dual disability

Hearing

Hearing is complicated. Sounds can be loud or soft, high or low, clear or "fuzzy" in quality. A hearing problem can involve a problem with one or all of these characteristics.

deafness and hard-of-hearing

There are several ways to define a hearing disability. *Deafness* means that a person has very severe hearing losses in both ears. These losses make it extremely difficult to learn and maintain language. *Hard-of-hearing* means that the person has some loss of hearing.

The location of damage also can define a hearing disability. Hearing depends on the passage of sound through a number of structures. When there is damage to the ear, ear drum, or middle ear, the person has a conduction loss. Generally, a hearing aid helps a conduction loss. When the damage is in the inner ear or auditory nerve, it is called sensorineural loss. About 5% of the general population have a hearing loss, but only one in 1,000 people is deaf.

Vision

There are many kinds of visual problems. People who have visual difficulties might be blind or partially sighted. *Blindness* and partial sightedness are words that are legally defined. This way, people with serious visual impairments can receive certain benefits.

These legal definitions are based on *visual acuity* and *peripheral vision.* When you look forward, peripheral vision is the range of vision on the sides. The degrees of a visual arc are used to measure peripheral vision.

People who are blind have little or no useful vision. Legally, blindness is defined two ways:

1. A person's central visual acuity is 20/200 or less in the better eye with the best possible correction. In other words, a person can recognize objects at a distance of twenty feet that a person with normal vision can recognize at 200 feet.

2. A person's peripheral vision is severely restricted to an angle no greater than twenty degrees. In other words, a person with this problem can see only a very limited area at one time.

Partially sighted people have visual acuity between 20/200 and 20/70 in the better eye with the best possible correction. Many people with visual impairments have some remaining vision. These are typical terms:

Myopia: nearsightedness

Hyperopia: farsightedness

Astigmatism: a condition that causes distorted images

Cataracts: a clouding of the lens of the eye causing blurred vision

Glaucoma: a buildup of fluid behind the eye

Many people have mild myopia or hyperopia. However, serious visual disabilities are rare. Only one in 1,000 people is legally blind, the same figure as for deafness.

blindness and partial sightedness

Other Kinds of Disabilities

There are far more kinds of disabilities than can be discussed in this manual. For example, some people may experience a variety of physical disabilities not already mentioned related to amputation, disease, a spinal cord or other motor injury, or some other cause. There are also health disorders such as diabetes, heart problems, asthma, cystic fibrosis, cancer, and AIDS. In addition, there are people who have various communication problems, including voice, language, and speech disorders. Again, while it is important to understand a person's disability and the challenges it presents, it is even more important to understand individuals and their capabilities and life goals.

A Brief History of Services

Throughout history, people have treated people with disabilities in inhumane ways. Older civilizations left children with disabilities to die by exposing them to the weather. Some kept them as "fools" for amusement. In the middle ages, people who were poor, elderly, or disabled were placed in local jails. When society began to build asylums, one perceived advantage was that it was cheaper to feed and house these individuals this way than to jail them or let them wander and depend on local charity.

In the 1800s, pioneers such as Itard, Seguin, and others began to demonstrate effective training techniques and founded residential training schools. By 1900, over 14,000 people were living in institutions, with the annual cost per resident only a few hundred dollars—a pitifully small amount of money for a year of care. Then came the rise of the eugenics movement in the early 1900s. This led to the advocacy of sterilization of the "feebleminded"

> "... the moron ... is a burden ... [and] is responsible to a large degree for many if not all of our social problems."
>
> – Dr. Henry Goddard, 1915

to improve the human race by "better breeding." Some believed that mental illness and mental retardation were completely genetic and caused many of society's problems, such as poverty, crime, and drunkenness.

People with disabilities became viewed by many as a menace. While these views subsided by the middle of the century, they were replaced by others that viewed disabilities as lifelong illness in need of special treatment, apart from society. The original goal of institutions, to change people with retardation into individuals of normal intelligence, shifted from education to long-term medical care and protection.

By 1967, nearly 195,000 people were in 108 public residential institutions, and the annual cost per resident had grown to nearly $3,000. As institutions grew in size, they became more focused on efficiency and control. Rigid rules were developed, personal possessions were not allowed, and residents were made to wear institutional clothing. After a while, it became obvious that the goal was not to protect people from the challenges of society, but rather to protect society from people with disabilities.

Growth of Community Services

By the 1960s, there were efforts to develop alternative services in local communities. Exposure of conditions and abuse led to public outrage and court involvement directing change. Research began to document the negative effects on development of life in an institution. By the 1970s, normalization and *deinstitutionalization* were becoming national priorities.

deinstitutionalization

In the 1980s, community services had taken hold as a viable alternative to institutions, and through the 1990s, the number of people who lived in institutions declined steadily. Annual costs, however, had risen to nearly $100,000 per resident per year. By 1997, just over 56,000 people with developmental disabilities remained in state-operated institutions, while only about 1,000 people with psychiatric disabilities were in state-run psychiatric institutions.

Despite people continuing to leave large state-run facilities, people with disabilities still, until very recently, were viewed as needing lifelong, systematic training in order to live successfully in the community and to be employable. As a result, services for people with severe disabilities were based on determining the best slot within a segregated human services system. This system trained people in building "readiness" for community life. It anticipated the individual would move from one program to another as he or she progressed. Movement and placement factors were determined through standardized evaluations of readiness and feasibility. Most services were developed around simulated rather than actual settings.

"My name is Russell Daniels. I was twelve when I was sent to a state school. When I left I was twenty-eight... I'm really proud to be out and I never want to go back to any institution at all... Now, I live like a king. I'm happy I do what I want, go where I want, I can come back when I want. I live by myself. I pay my own rent. I pay my bills. I work at the Senior Center. I love it. And they all love me."

Russell Daniels,
board member of the self-advocacy
organization Open Door Club,
Belchertown, MA
Parallels in Time,
MN Governor's Council on Developmental Disabilities

Growth of Supported Living

One outcome of these readiness-based approaches was that few people ever really got the chance to live a normal community life. As these community program models began to be viewed as problematic in the 1980s, both people with disabilities and disability professionals began to develop new ideas. These approaches, supported living, supported employment, and supported recreation, tried to support each person with a disability to live, work, and recreate in regular community settings of his or her choosing.

They are based on the idea of *inclusion*, or being a part of the mainstream of life. Inclusion can mean many things, such as attending neighborhood schools, working at a job in a career of one's choice, and living in a place one truly could call home. These ideas focus on providing training and supports in community settings in ways that are natural to the setting. And the people who use the services are the ones who set their direction.

inclusion

These new programs have expanded—thanks to recent court decisions, legislation, and changes in funding and policy. Together they all have contributed to more normalized and life-enhancing services. The Americans with Disabilities Act, for instance, has removed many barriers to employment, transportation, and accessibility to public places.

Growth of Self-Determination and Self-Advocacy

The coming years likely will see the continued growth of *self-determination* by people with disabilities. Self-determination is a term that means that people with disabilities control the decisions that affect their lives. This means many things about how people with disabilities live, and how services are provided to them. For instance, self-determination means:

self-determination

- having full citizenship by participating with all his or her related rights in community life
- being able to make an informed choice about how, where, and with whom to live, work, and play
- having control of the processes and the resources that will be invested in their lives

Having full citizenship, informed choice, and control of resources translates to a new and different system of disability services. It is one in which the person, with his or her chosen family, friends, and advocates, obtains direct access to funding for those services and supports needed to be a full community member and citizen. The person can then choose, with appropriate safeguards, how to spend that money for his or her chosen lifestyle, whether it is for support from a disability agency or from somewhere else.

The obstacles to realizing such a system are many. As a result, over the past few years, there has been a tremendous growth in *self-advocacy* by people with disabilities. Self-advocates are people with

self-advocacy

disabilities themselves speaking out. They are acting as leaders to promote self-determination and community integration. They are also tackling tough issues, like the continued segregation of people, high unemployment rates, discrimination, and inadequate or inappropriate rules, laws, and funding.

This movement can be traced back to the 1960s, when Benjt Nirje, director of the Swedish Association for Persons with Mental Retardation, organized a club where people with mental retardation met to experience "normal" community activities. He said, "This is akin to any decent revolt... This struggle for respect and independence is always the normal way to obtain personal dignity and a sense of liberty and equality." These clubs eventually led to several national conferences, including one in the US. In 1974, nearly 600 self-advocates from across the US attended the first US conference of "People First." By 1995, there were over 600 self-advocacy organizations in the US, cutting across all kinds of disabilities to advocate for self-determination, political power, and civil rights.

Despite this, controversy remains in many places over the future system of service for people with disabilities. What's more, the historical practice of institutionalization has led to two trends that unfortunately still persist in today's services:

- grouping together large numbers of people with disabilities
- distancing services away from communities

> **The development of institutions led to two trends that persist even today:**
> - **Grouping persons with disabilities**
> - **Distancing services away from local communities**

Summary

People with disabilities are individuals first. They are people with diverse skills, dreams, aptitudes, and life experiences. Understanding different types of disabilities and their causes can be useful in beginning to understand the challenges someone may have. But **ultimately it is your personal relationship with each person as an individual that best will help you to enhance his or her life. This includes awareness of each person's dreams and goals, the skills and resources you both have, and your knowledge of the community and its people.**

Labels and the Meaning of Progress

"I was born in a family of three brothers and five sisters in a little town. I was the only one labeled retarded, because my parents somehow thought that I was different. What they didn't understand is that everybody is different in some ways. But in other ways we all have the same needs.

We all need to know that we are loved ... I didn't have special needs, I had common needs. Everybody needs to be hugged, everybody needs to know that they can communicate within the family circle. Everybody needs to know that they can have friends next door ... that they can have a good education and that people are not deciding their education for them.

I went to a totally segregated school ... And all I did all day was to figure out crossword puzzles, how to use a coloring book, and how to print my name—I never learned to write my name, because people thought that I could not progress that far.

Well, let me tell you something about progress ... A lot of people who aren't valued in this system have to go through life very lonely, very oppressed—if they live that long. And people call it progress. I do not call that progress...

I have been institutionalized, because I did not have anywhere else to go in the community. What is the importance of community— what do we mean by community if community is not there to support or to make a commitment to love?"

– Pat Worth
"The Importance of Speaking for Yourself"
Address to The Association for Persons with Severe Handicaps

1. What are some ways a label can be harmful to a person? Give an example.

2. Understanding a person's disability is useful, but to assist an individual best, you need to:
   - a. test the person
   - b. know their IQ score
   - c. get to know the person well
   - d. find a specialized program

3. People tend to act in ways which we assume they should act. This is called
_____. How can this work <u>positively</u> for a person?

4. One alternative to assigning people a disability label is to look at how well their functional behaviors support their chosen lifestyle. Give an example of a functional behavior and how it might impact on a life goal, such as "living in an apartment on my own."

5. Describe one way of defining mental retardation, and give an example.

6. Mental retardation is often confused with mental illness. Describe how they are different.

7. Give two examples of the inhumane treatment people with disabilities experienced in the past. Describe the alternatives for services available today.

8. Legal blindness is determined by which two measurements:
   a. visual acuity   c. myopia
   b. glaucoma   d. peripheral vision

9. People with epilepsy often experience changes in the normal brain rhythms which cause _____. In what ways might this cause functional difficulties?

10. The most important person(s) in determining how services should be provided is/are:
   a. the executive director   c. the case manager/support coordinator
   b. direct service staff   d. the person with a disability and his or her family

Part B

A Quality Life in the Community

Normalization is . . .
using supports, experiences, learning strategies, and environments that promote positive relationships, personal behaviors, and individual characteristics and roles that a community will value in a person.

social role valorization

During the early 1960s, several American educators travelled to the Scandinavian region to experience firsthand how people with disabilities lived there. After visiting several locations, they were surprised and impressed with what they saw. People with disabilities were living in ordinary homes in the community, cooking meals, going to work or school, and making their own choices about their lives.

This would have been startling to any professional from this country from that era. We had a long philosophy and history of services that kept many people with disabilities separated from their homes, families, and communities. Yet here were people living according to a philosophy called "*normalization.*" The realization that people with disabilities, when provided with the right support and opportunities, could live as we all do began a social movement in this country as well.

By 1972, Wolf Wolfensberger had become North America's leader in normalization, or as it is now called, *social role valorization* (SRV). This concept refers to both a philosophy and a policy in working with people with disabilities. It states that people who have disabilities are entitled **to decide among options of living that everybody else has in their community.** In particular, people should be supported to pursue **lifestyles of their choosing that enhance their status.** This means they have the right to a home, a career, and recreational pursuits like others in their community, and they have the right to express themselves as individuals in following these lifestyles.

To assure these rights, most service systems use normalization and SRV as a basic philosophy. Many state standards require policies and procedures that support normalization. This way, people with disabilities should have better opportunities to enjoy patterns of life and conditions of everyday living that other people experience.

> When we understand what perpetuates myths, we can work to change them. One of the most powerful ways is for persons with disabilities to participate successfully in their communities—as good neighbors, good workers, and good friends to those around them.

myths about disability

However, **required policies do not always translate into reality**. There are numerous obstacles to obtaining a valued lifestyle. Having a disability in our society means that most people will think of you as different in a negative way. Our culture values being productive, skilled, attractive, and affluent. For a number of reasons that have little to do with the people themselves, these attributes rarely are connected to people who are disabled. Rather, they often are wrongly perceived as people who are incompetent, "funny-looking" children who never grow up, or as even dangerous or sickly.

These perceptions are myths. Children with disabilities grow into adults with needs of interdependence, privacy, accomplishment, sexuality, and responsibility. Individuals with disabilities can learn a diverse range of valued skills. They have demonstrated their on-the-job productivity and their ability to manage a home, given the right supports. Although a disability can make one's appearance "different" from the norm, a more important reason some people with disabilities look different is because they have never been taught grooming or styles, the programs in which they find themselves are demeaning, or the people helping them do not think appearance is important.

Yet the myths are powerful. There has been much controversy in the United States surrounding some very basic issues for people with disabilities. Some neighborhoods have fought against people with disabilities living in their midst. Some people say they are uncomfortable having their children attend school with students with disabilities, or shopping in their communities alongside consumers with disabilities, or being near co-workers with disabilities.

The history of professional services often has supported these myths. By segregating people, by grouping people together, by labelling people, by creating "special institutions or special schools," we have made individuals appear even more different.

At the same time, services and attitudes are changing for the better. Part of the reason is a greater awareness of the principles of normalization. We also are learning how to better communicate with and educate the public about the rights of citizens with disabilities. And one of the most powerful ways to change attitudes is for people to participate successfully in their communities—as good neighbors, good workers, and good friends to those around them.

A big part of our job, then, is to understand how perceptions of people with disabilities are influenced, and to then support more valued social roles for people.

> *"The normalization principle reminds us of two things. First, just because a person has a negatively valued characteristic does not mean that we are justified in isolating him or her from community life. Second, the services we offer should attempt to balance personal characteristics which are seen negatively with others which are seen positively.*
>
> *A person labelled 'severely retarded' who has major mobility and speech problems (all characteristics which will change very slowly) presents a positive image if she or he is fashionably dressed, lives in an apartment with a roommate and a personal attendant, and is productively employed wiring electronic circuit boards...*
>
> *All of these characteristics—appearance, activities, living place, occupation—can be substantially influenced by the service system. The principle of normalization expects a service agency to increase people's positive characteristics."*
>
> John O'Brien, *The Principle of Normalization*

Normalization does not emphasize how people with disabilities are **different** from others. Clearly, we are all different in certain ways. But at the same time, we are all more alike as people with the same needs and rights.

- It stresses what each person **can do rather than what he or she can't do.**
- It places an emphasis on the **environment** and the experiences encountered.
- It supports people to **follow their own interests** leading to being a worker, neighbor, and friend to others.

> **We must work to reduce the grouping of persons with disabilities, and design services that are integrated and individualized.**

- It assumes that all people can **learn**. Therefore, experiences can be planned that foster growth and learning.

When you plan and develop services for an individual, there are a number of considerations that can enhance his or her status and provide an opportunity to develop meaningful relationships and valued social roles. Among these are supporting individuality; helping the person acquire skills and competencies; helping to provide positive settings where people will live, work, and recreate; avoiding giving subtle negative messages through language, postures, and interactions; facilitating community relationships; and supporting rhythms and routines within positive and prestigious social roles.

Supporting Self-Determination

You can be a source of support for self-determination, that is, helping people with disabilities making choices about their lives and their services. One of the main obstacles people face to self-determination is a perception by others of their limited competence. This can lead to limited choices or being offered choices that are not meaningful. For example, a person with a disability may be offered one choice and given the opportunity to say only "yes" or "no."

Sometimes alternatives are pre-selected and presented without complete information "to make it easier for the person to choose." While some people may have difficulty with too much information, rather than limiting choices it is better to provide training to people with disabilities on how to make meaningful choices. We should also provide extra time and assistance for people to discover their own preferences and look at the full range of options.

Advocate Michael Smull has noted that helping people make choices includes three parts: understanding preference, providing opportunities, and respecting people's control over the process. Preferences are not only what someone likes but also his or her desires and hopes for the future. You need to learn who people want to spend time with, what they want to do during that time, and where they want to spend their time. Control is being able to make decisions about opportunities to fulfill preferences. Some ways you can help support self-determination include:

choice-making

> "Preferences are what people want. Opportunities are what is available. Control is the authority to use an opportunity to satisfy a preference."
> — Michael Smull

- Start all planning with a "blank slate," free from assumptions.
- Help people to express their preferences.
- Help people search out as many options as possible when they are faced with decisions.
- Do not be limited by "what already exists" or the "quickest solution."
- Explore fully each possibility.
- Help people to make their choices and express their decisions.
- When people must compromise, be sure to let everyone know clearly that they have made a compromise.

Supporting Individual Lifestyles

When people with disabilities are grouped together for "treatment" in a facility-based program, it becomes extremely difficult for them to be perceived as individuals in their own right. The group becomes labelled as different, and services are developed around the group's needs rather than each individual.

People's needs tend to revolve around relationships, quality homes, and good jobs. To meet each individual's needs, each network of resources will be unique. We must work to reduce the grouping of people with disabilities, and design services that are integrated and individualized.

Individuality can have a powerful effect on improving self-image and esteem. When Susan began a job in an office downtown, she met many new friends, took more care about her appearance, and took greater pride in her new role in her company. The people around her saw her as "Susan," and not as one of a larger group. They treated her with respect for her work.

People with disabilities will not be valued for their uniqueness as long as they travel, shop, recreate, work, and live in self-contained groups. Supporting individuality will help to change self-perceptions from a person who is dependent to one who is a responsible and singular citizen of the community.

Building Competencies

Besides living in a community environment, individuals will benefit by learning skills that help them to participate fully in their community and to be interdependent. These skills can help an individual to be more competent in his or her environment. For example, when Roger learns skills to do his job at the post office better, he is more likely to obtain a better paying, long-term, higher status position. The more competencies and skills a person possesses, the more choices a person will have in improving her or his image and status.

Feeding yourself, ordering from a menu, working productively, and taking the bus to town are examples of behaviors that help us participate in the everyday world. When you model and help someone learn skills such as these, you provide the tools to enhance capability and status, and ultimately help that person to lead a better life.

It is important to model and help people learn behaviors that allow them to fit smoothly into the community. The skills people learn should be physically adaptive and also socially enhancing.

> It is important to model and teach behaviors that will help people to participate fully in their community.

For example, a person should learn not only how to walk, but also how to walk with as normal a gait as possible; not only how to dress, but how to dress stylishly for age, situation, and season.

People with disabilities do have challenges that society must recognize and understand. A good example of this is the need for barrier-free environments. Yet, at the same time, people should not be overprotected. This may lead to unnecessary dependency. So if an individual wants to learn to cook, he or she should learn to prepare meals with whatever technology and support we can provide. This is true for all skills that result in more independent living. Overprotection can slow growth for any person.

Learning skills such as these should occur in the context of real situations. Adults with disabilities often have spent their whole lives "getting ready" for a job or "getting ready" for living in the community. **The best way to learn functional skills is in real jobs, homes, or communities**, and not in readiness programs.

Valued Community Settings

The location, type, and arrangement of a person's physical environment helps determine the kind of life he or she leads. Housing, for instance, should be truly a home in a neighborhood of choice. It should reflect personal preferences for decor and function, rather than functioning as a "program center." This also includes a right to privacy and a right to property. Each person in her or his own home has possessions, clothing, and money. If a person has chosen to share a room, then a separate, personal, and safe place should be available to keep private things.

> **The signals a program sends will have a powerful, long-term effect on public attitudes toward people with disabilities. If a goal is to increase community participation of people who may be seen as different, the message sent by what we do is as important as what we accomplish.**

A person might need assistance in determining the decor and function of rooms. Attractive furniture, curtains, plants, and pictures are also important. For example, tastefully arranged living room furniture creates a homey feel, while office furniture will give an impression of a program.

People also should work, learn, or recreate in typical community environments. Unfortunately, some programs that serve adults still group people in segregated settings. They may even utilize materials or decorations that are more typically found in an elementary school. For example, children's toys and games and childish holiday decorations have the effect of conveying to others that these individuals are thought of as children. This is harmful for an individual who needs to be seen as a competent adult.

Efforts should always be made to respect individual preferences while working to enhance settings and environments. Opportunities for choice and selection should be a part of designing personal space. We should be striving to help **add status** and desirability to people's homes, workplaces, and transportation.

Respectful Interaction

The interactions you have with the people whom you support are tremendously important. These interactions should be a blend of professionalism and personal respect. You need to use good judgement as you choose moments to teach or correct as well as when you choose moments to provide support. You need to respect the preferences and decisions made by the individuals with whom you work regarding what they want and need.

Interactions involve your words, your tone, and the loudness of your voice, as well as your facial expressions and gestures. You should try to communicate in ways that fit the situation. Adults who respect one another do not refer to each other by labels, derogatory nicknames, or stereotypes. Nor do they act as a parent. Rather, they value people who communicate with them **as peers in respectful ways.** How we interact tells the world a lot about how we view the people we are with.

> The language we use in working with persons with disabilities can be a powerful force. The names we choose for our programs can convey capability or pity. The way we address people says a lot about how we feel about them. Always strive to enhance each person's image and skills. Take care of how you dress, speak, and portray people.

Enhancing Appearance

Our appearance also conveys a message to others. How we dress and how we present ourselves in our jobs portray what we think of our job as well as our opinion of people with disabilities. Dress should be appropriate to circumstances, but we should strive to **model an enhancing appearance** that others may appreciate. This is as much true of ourselves as it is true for people who have disabilities. People are far more likely to be respected when they present an appealing appearance.

Developing Rhythms and Routines

Most of us conduct our days, weeks, and years in a comfortable pattern. *Routines* are the particular activities we go through each day and week. *Rhythms* are the periodic, predictable changes that occur over time in our environments and our lives. Rhythms and routines are related. They often reflect our accommodation to changes in our world.

Many routines and rhythms are dictated by our society. People who do not follow them often are viewed as different. This is not to say that we must all follow the strict expectations of our culture as if we are robots. But we must understand how people become perceived negatively, and what helps to change those perceptions. People with disabilities should be supported to be unique, but also

patterns of community life

to learn the ways the community and culture will value or devalue their uniqueness.

Like all of us, people with disabilities should have the opportunity to maintain **patterns of living that reflect a normal rhythm** of the day, week, and season. Adults typically rise and retire at "normal" times, eat three meals approximately five hours apart, go to work, and choose their own leisure or recreational activities and friends. Seasonal changes should reflect variety in types of food, clothing, and leisure activities pursued, as preferred by each person's chosen lifestyle.

Helping to Develop a Network of Relationships

> "We need to belong intimately to a few people who are permanent elements in our lives. A life without people, without ... people who belong to us, people who will be there for us, people who need us and whom we need in return, may be very rich in other things, but in human terms, it is no life at all; ... all the complicated structures we ... create, are built on sand. Only our relationships to other people endure."
>
> – Harold Kushner
> *When All You've Ever Wanted Isn't Enough*

Most people feel that the key to a quality life in the community rests on relationships. Our friends, families, neighbors, and acquaintances are important people in our lives. Even in our work, our co-workers influence our success. Research has shown that a significant factor for job satisfaction is to have strong social relationships there.

Sometimes a staff person becomes a long-term friend to someone with whom they work. But it is just as important to **support the development of diverse relationships with the rich variety of people** in a person's community. We can facilitate this by providing introductions and opening up our own networks of relationships. We can also help people develop shared experiences, gain access to social organizations, and participate in typical community activities. Some of these types of relationships are described next.

Personal and Family Relationships

At the inner core of our social life are the relationships we deeply value. These could include our life partner, children and parents, brothers and sisters, boyfriend or girlfriend, or closest friends. The bonds we have with some of these people are more intimate, and we tend to reveal more of our private selves in our interactions with these people.

Being a valued family member, for instance, provides reciprocal bonds of love and support. Parents lovingly guide a son and daughter, and children bring parents pride and joy. Siblings, grandparents, cousins, and others can provide a network of family support where "blood is thicker than water." It is often our family we turn to in times of trouble or celebration.

Adults with disabilities have the same adult needs for these personal relationships as everyone else does. This includes sexual intimacy as well. All people experience sexual feelings, and human sexuality can be expressed in different ways. Many adults with disabilities will need support and guidance in developing personal relationships of this nature. These relationships also carry personal responsibilities, mutual desire and consent, and a need for educated decisions about actions that affect those a person is close to.

Staff responsibilities in this area can be complex, and a discussion of them is beyond the scope of this manual. What is important is to recognize and respect each individual's personal lifestyle choices in the social arena. Obtain guidance from your supervisor and the individual himself or herself in how to help guide and support personal relationships.

Joining a Community

There is a lot of confusion about what "community" is and is not. Community refers to people participating and **sharing life together through mutual support in various ways in localities and circles of interest.** But communities are diverse and not always coherent. They can be formal or informal, large or small, singular or plural.

Community is not a "training environment," nor should it be foreign territory for human services workers. It is common to hear about a person with a disability "in the community," when he or she is actually very lonely and isolated.

Community means active participation and sharing. To facilitate this, we should help connect people into communities and build communities around people. This is done best when you know the sometimes hidden resources a community offers, and you can assist people to gain access to them. Some ideas to do this include:

- Find people with common interests.
- Build familiarity with local businesses.
- Join associations and clubs.
- Become recognized in your neighborhood.
- Seek gathering places.
- Find people who can provide introductions.
- Create gatherings.
- Give something to the community.
- Utilize existing networks.

the intimacy of family and friends

communities provide mutual support

"One of the more important things that has helped me get to a more balanced place is my "circle of support." It's sometimes easier to talk about what circles are not than to say exactly what they are. They're not group therapy, and they're not part of a program or another treatment modality. It's not something that's forced on anyone, or something that has a formula or outline or steps or stages. It's not an intervention written onto someone's rehabilitation plan.

Circles are "run" by the person with the disability. That person decides who the people are in his or her life that have given support, the people to trust and rely on who have some investment in helping him or her achieve goals. Then the focus person decides the who, what, when, where, how, and why of the circle, and the circle is created. "

— J. Alyson Hastings
Voices in the Storm

- Support family networks.
- Attend civic meetings.
- Use public recreational facilities.

Circles of Support

A *circle of support* is a group of people who meet regularly to help a person with a disability accomplish personal goals. The members of a circle of support usually include friends, family members, co-workers, neighbors, and sometimes service providers. The majority of people are not paid to be there — they are involved because they care about the person and have made a commitment to work together on his or her behalf. While circles do not exclude paid service providers, the majority of members are non-paid, typical community people. The circle thus depends on the local community for its effectiveness.

Advocacy from the Community

Many people with disabilities, either due to their experiences, the reactions of others to them, or the nature of their disability, have not been able to initiate or develop those things they wish to have happen for themselves. This includes friendships, going to activities and events of interest, or accessing services or supports.

The concept of *citizen advocacy* embraces the idea that people with disabilities can gain help in personal life goals by being connected to someone through friendship and companionship. That connection can help spark access to areas of interest in ways professional human services and sometimes even family cannot.

citizen advocacy

A citizen advocate, sometimes referred to as a *community connector,* is someone who is already well connected to the social networks of a given community. He or she is unpaid and independent of human services. This person gets to know someone with a disability through spending time and doing things together. He or she then works to understand, respond to, and represent the person's interests.

Some states and localities have formal citizen advocacy programs, while others may support the idea informally as part of other services, such as support coordination or case management. There are numerous things a citizen advocate can help obtain or provide:

- Introduce the individual to other people who share the same interests.
- Help the individual find job leads.
- Support the person in times of trouble.
- Celebrate accomplishments and special events with the person.
- Just spend time together.
- Go to places to do things of mutual interest.
- Sponsor the person into social networks.
- Help the person become a member of civic and other local organizations.
- Talk over life's events to make sense of the past and make plans for the future.
- Advocate and help plan with the person the nature of future services and supports.

Planning for the Future

For a person to realize a rich life within the fabric of a community, some planning is necessary. One of the most effective approaches to such planning is called *person-centered planning*, or *personal futures planning*. In this process, a team of people who care about the person come together. This team, which sometimes becomes a circle of support, then works with the person to explore and determine his or her resources and life dreams.

personal futures planning

It is then the team's task to organize all available resources to help the person move toward that future. Your participation in planning teams such as this can be powerful. It is an opportunity to first of all listen and learn about the individual in new ways. Then, as part of a group process with the person at the center, you can determine what your support role should be.

Person-centered strategies focus on a person's ability rather than deficits. The approach is to build a vision of the future about how that person wants to live and work, along with his or her social relationships, hobbies and leisure activities, settings, and lifestyle. To provide support for some-

> One of the greatest opportunities you have to support a person with a disability is to listen, learn, and help him or her plan a life for the future.

one, we first need to ask about the life dreams and motivations that contribute to this individual's personality. As the answers come together, they will direct the development of a plan so that the person's vision of life becomes a reality.

A Home and a Job of One's Own

Two of the most important things that either connect people with disabilities to others in community life or set them apart is how they live and work. All people, including those who have disabilities, should be able to have a good job they enjoy and a home to call their own.

A Real Job

Adults with disabilities all should have job opportunities in community settings. This is important for many reasons. A job provides self-sufficiency. The wages from a job can support a chosen lifestyle, buying the things a person likes, wants, or needs. Money earned enables a person to vacation, go to the movies, or to have fun in other ways.

> **Recent federal legislative changes state that all people with disabilities are presumed able to be employed.**

Beyond money, work brings self-esteem, respect from others, and a sense of accomplishment and personal growth. Making friends is another thing that happens at work. We already have discussed the importance of meeting and developing friendships with all kinds of people. Relationships provide needed support and stability.

Real jobs can be thought of in many different ways. The different kinds of people who are present in a workplace should be similar to what exists throughout that community. There shouldn't be an unnatural grouping of people with disabilities working together just to make support or supervision easier. A real job also provides pay for work that is necessary, rather than just practice work. Wages should reflect what people accomplish and be the same as what others make for doing the same type of work. An employee with a real job is respected for his or her contribution as part of a work team—there is dignity and status in participating.

Unfortunately, most adults with disabilities remain unemployed or underemployed. This is partly the result of a slowly changing service system that keeps people getting ready for work rather than helping to develop meaningful jobs as quickly as possible.

supported employment

There are many ways of helping an individual find, keep, and advance in a job. *Supported employment* refers to giving ongoing services to assist people, regardless of how severe their disability, to be employed in a community business. This service has come packaged in many models, each with advantages and disadvantages. Rather than trying to help an individual by fitting him or her into any one vocational model or program, it is more effective to help each person pursue his or her interests and skills toward an individual job.

A Real Home

A home is a place to express one's individual personality. This is because it is a place where a person is loved. It is where a person feels secure. Home is also where there is a freedom of choice, within reason, about how to express oneself. And this expression can take place in a wide variety of ways. For instance, the kind of neighborhood, setting, house and color, landscaping, furniture, and even style of housekeeping tells others about who lives in a home. Whether through home ownership or renting, the person should truly make the home his or her own, rather than residing in a program that includes housing.

elements of a good home life

Yet this basic human need for a good, affordable home is often hard to meet. In particular, adults with disabilities often lack the money, support, or community connections to have a place of their own. As a result, they may be limited to living choices that are pre-designed housing models. These models usually limit individualized expression.

For a residence to be truly a personal home, it should match what a person wants, needs, and can reasonably afford. This can be provided through a concept called *supported living*. As in employment, supported living services begin by exploring each person's capabilities, interests, resources, and social connections. From there, staff help the person look at where and how he or she wants to live.

supported living

A good place to start is to consider the kind of neighborhood a person prefers. A neighborhood is a small community tied together by geography, people, shared building styles, or something else such as values or attitudes. By thinking about what an ideal neighborhood would look like, you can help the individual create a vision to guide housing decisions. The person also should consider how and with whom he or she wishes to live. Some people enjoy having roommates. Others may prefer to live on their own or to remain with their family for now.

Finally, the person might need ongoing support for different aspects of home life. This could include cooking, cleaning, laundry, and choosing furniture. Assistance might occur through training, giving advice, or helping to adapt the setting.

Associational Life

People in communities come together for reasons other than where they live or work. There are formal and informal associations, for example, that are based on commonalities, such as groups for elderly citizens, artists, sports, charitable organizations, collectors, computer users, health groups, service groups, and so on. These groups tend to have great continuity and a large capacity for shared support for those who belong. Says author John McKnight, *"Once we have understood the nature of the community of associations that is the center of our democracy, we can begin to consider those methods that lead to excluded people being incorporated into this community life."* Thus, an important way people with disabilities can be a part of their community is by joining associations that interest them.

Recreation

Recreation is another important part of community life, where one can meet friends who share common interests, learn new things, and improve one's health. Some of the problems people with disabilities experience in participating in recreation reflects the same barriers they experience in employment and housing. They can be stereotyped as children needing overprotection, discriminated against and offered segregated activities that they attend with other people with disabilities or with people who do not correspond to their age. For people to enjoy and grow from their leisure activities, keep the following in mind:

- The activity should be age-appropriate; the individual should find people in his or her age group also in attendance.
- The activity should include a diversity of people, rather than be limited to people with disabilities.
- The activity should be one the person has interest in or one in which the person is exploring his or her interest.
- The setting should be accessible for maximum participation of the individual.
- Any supports the individual receives to participate should be as natural, non-intrusive, and non-stigmatizing as possible.

Spiritual Life

Another association that people with disabilities should have access to is the community of faith of their choice. Regularly attending a place of worship and being with others who share one's faith is an important part of life for many people, as well as a valued social role in most communities. Many congregations also offer community service and social activities.

community associations

Summary

There are many obstacles people with disabilities face when trying to live a valued community life. This is why your **judgement** is so important about what supports will be helpful and what won't. Often, professionals use their own standards of choice as a yardstick for what is appropriate. But this doesn't always work well. Each person is unique. In addition, **a person with a disability has a negative label and is already at risk** of rejection, segregation, and limited opportunity. For someone already faced with this, we need to be even more conscious of settings, appearances, language, social roles, and behavior than the yardsticks we use for ourselves.

Valued people in our culture who don't choose to dress or act in the mainstream might be viewed as eccentric or individualistic. But someone who is already "devalued" likely will find themselves even more labeled as deviant. Understanding each of these patterns helps define positive practices. This will ensure that people with disabilities experience dignity, individual respect, and age-appropriate settings and practices. They should also have opportunities to pursue valued social roles through where they work, live, and recreate in their communities.

Vision of the Future

"If it were all in place, if people had all that they want and need... You would live with your family until you grew up. Then you would choose where to live next and with whom to live.

Often the help you needed would come out of friendship, neighborliness, familial concern, or love. You would return the favors... Some kinds of help you might need indefinitely, while others would last only for an evening. Sometimes the help would come to you at home, sometimes you would go to it. You would have a choice in the services no matter where you live, and if you were not happy you could make a change.

As an adult, you might get further education or you might go to work. You would choose work you wanted to spend your life at and while you might have several false starts, you would receive the training necessary to help you begin.

If you were ever called by any names other than the one your parents gave you, they would be terms of affection or praise. The way you were different would be thought a natural and true thing. All the colors of life would be appreciated equally, not just the blues and reds and greens of intellect, appearance, and monetary worth ..."

– Everyday Lives
Pennsylvania Department of Public Welfare

A Quality Life in the Community

POSTSESSION REVIEW

Name _____   Agency _____
Program _____   Trainer_____
Date _____   Score _____

1. People with disabilities have the same life goals as all people do. But in our culture, someone with a disability is at risk of being perceived negatively. Name three attributes that would promote a positive image for someone with a disability.

2. Choose one myth about people with disabilities and explain why it isn't true.

3. Choose one person you have met who has a disability and has experienced success in their community. Describe what contributed to her or his success. Cite at least two things.

4. In order for people with disabilities to fit smoothly into the community, it is important to
   _____ (choose two).
   a. be sure they will "behave"
   b. teach functional skills
   c. be prepared for the worst
   d. always travel in groups
   e. ride in a van
   f. go bowling daily
   g. know their neighborhood and neighbors
   h. spend their day in a segregated building

5. What's troubling about this statement?
   "The mentally retarded should be protected by using sheltered facilities, particularly for the more severe ones."

6. Check the attributes that would promote a person's image.

    __ good appearance   __ traveling as a group in a van

    __ living in an eight-person group home   __ owning a home

    __ visiting friends   __ making $.52 per hour

    __ working at a local business   __ sharing a room with two other people

    __ learning to sort by color   __ attending social events specifically for people with disabilities

7. When people with disabilities wear well-fitting, stylish clothes, in what ways will their appearance affect their lives?

8. Name three things you could do in order to promote participation and friendships for Bob Johnson, a 40-year-old man who enjoys cooking, music, and being outdoors. Mr. Johnson is a person who likes meeting new people, uses a wheelchair, and is labelled as severely retarded.

9. When people with disabilities do things together as a group, they are more likely to be seen as valued individuals. True or false. Why?

10. Choose any that apply. People with disabilities have the right to:

    a. grow up   d. have sexual relationships

    b. live in the community   e. have a variety of friends

    c. work at a meaningful job   f. vote

Part C
Understanding and Supporting Effective Behavior

norms of behavior

In order to support someone in his or her pursuit of a quality life in the community, it is crucial to have an understanding of community expectations of behavior. Behavior is what people do. It is our observable actions such as smiling, talking, eating, and dressing. People constantly behave, and we each perform an enormous number of behaviors each day.

Certain environments and situations have rules and norms of public behavior. For example, at a grocery store, it is expected that people will browse quietly, make selections, and pay for their purchases at cash registers when they have completed shopping. There are similar rules in a post office, at a bank, at a concert, or on a job.

Besides the rules for different places, there are also expectations for situations. When we meet someone new, for instance, it is expected that we shake hands, smile, and perhaps say a social pleasantry. If someone has angered us, there are limits on what reactions are socially acceptable and what behaviors are not.

Sometimes these standards of acting can be complex, unclear, or unspoken. Some rules are informal, while others are mandated by laws or regulations. When someone does not understand expectations of behavior, or fails to conform to them, his or her actions will likely limit the opportunity for success, participation, status, and friendship. As discussed in Part B, these are important things in order to be seen as a valued member of a community.

Meeting norms for social behavior helps people to participate as valued members of their community.

The rest of this section discusses basic information about behavior, what influences our actions, and useful techniques to change what we do. But it is very important to realize that this information must be applied with respect and in the context of helping people with disabilities realize their goals for careers, home life, relationships, and other aspects of community living.

Behavior as Communication

Because some people with disabilities have difficulty communicating, behavior can inform us about how they are feeling or thinking. We always should ask questions about what each person's behavior may be **communicating**.

Behavior that breaks social norms can be challenging for a staff person to respond to. But these actions also provide clues about how people may **feel** about their jobs, their homes, or the tasks at hand. Or it could signal other things. For example, there may be a medical or emotional condition of which we are unaware. There are instances of people who were made to follow restrictive behavior programs for self-injury, only to discover later that they acted because they were in pain from a physical problem, such as a tooth abscess or stomach ulcer.

There may be other factors to consider as well. For example, a possible source of discontent is when our home or job unexpectedly changes in ways we don't like. We may become bored, disgruntled, or frustrated very easily. Generally, it is not too long before we exercise some control and begin to wish for something different.

If forced to stay, we may try to exert control in another way. And that might be by our behavior. Boredom, for example, can lead to many kinds of actions to alleviate the feeling of unending time. We create games, cause trouble with others, or do other kinds of things to interest ourselves.

Still another issue involves having a simple personality conflict. We have all had the experience of not getting along with someone at work. This can cause all sorts of performance and related behavioral problems. When our behavior breaks expected work norms because of social or work pressures, we can find ourselves in trouble with our co-workers or our supervisor.

As you can see, having behavior challenges is not an issue just for people with disabilities. We are all susceptible to breaking social norms with our actions. Some of us have simply learned better coping responses, or even are simply better at not getting caught!

This illustrates that people behave for many different reasons. While most behavior is learned from environments, there are other internal factors as well. Changing behavior is complex and can occur in many ways. Because much of the behavior people express is

> Professionals often develop behavior programs in immediate response to an "undesirable behavior." Often we do not ask enough important questions about what the person's behavior really means. Since some persons with disabilities have difficulty communicating, behavior may be their primary way of telling us things. Challenging behavior that we often call "inappropriate" may well say a lot about what a person *feels* about a job, home, or task.

learned, it is important to realize that our behaviors are not fixed. We can learn new behaviors, unlearn old ones, and change the things we do.

Analyzing Behavior

Helping someone change ineffective or unwelcome behavior begins with a thorough understanding of the individual's past and present, hopes and desires for the future, relationships with others, and the norms of the setting. Behavior analysis is a way to examine and then help a person to change or learn new behaviors. It has become one of the most widely used techniques in the fields of education and training. It provides an opportunity to improve behaviors so that people can function more effectively, enjoy a wider range of experiences, and enhance their relationships with others.

Because behavior analysis involves a set of procedures that reduces complex problems to individualized learnable bits, it allows a person to build up a sequence of behaviors that together make up a social "skill." But a skill is not just a simple behavior chain. Learning the rules about when or when not to exercise certain behaviors, and under what conditions, is a difficult learning challenge for anyone.

guard against oversimplification

For example, the risk in reducing complex behavior includes a tendency to oversimplify or misinterpret situations. On the basis of a very limited amount of information, we often jump to conclusions about the nature of "the problem." But behavioral analysis requires careful consideration. Behavior is influenced by the environment and environments are very complicated. Factors such as health; state of hunger or thirst; comfort, mood, or attentiveness; background lighting, noise, and temperature; and history of experiences all play a part in why a person behaves or reacts in certain ways.

Observable Actions

In order to be more precise when analyzing behavior, begin by describing what someone is doing using **clear and concrete** language. For instance, instead of saying Bob was *"upset,"* clearly state what it was that Bob did and the conditions around the action. (*"Bob cried as he left the room after reading the note."*) People think and have feelings, but there is no way to directly observe a feeling or a thought. We can only infer the way people feel and think by the way they act or by what they tell us. Actions can be observed. When we explain behavior, we describe what people do.

concrete language to describe behavior

Behavior is influenced by the environment, but any environment is more complicated than we realize. Many factors such as a person's health; state of hunger or thirst; comfort, mood, or attentiveness; background lighting; noise; temperature; and history of experiences play a part in why a person reacts in certain ways.

Sometimes when we infer how a person feels or thinks, we might use labels like "upset" as a shorthand to describe a set of behaviors. If we say "John is smart" or "Jane is angry," we actually stereotype their behavior. When we use a negative description such as "aggressive," we will have certain negative expectations about how the person will behave. Having expectations for aggression can set up conditions in which a person might play the role everyone expects, and aggression actually can become more likely. This does not help a person to learn new ways of behaving and can even prevent change.

If we avoid labelling, inferring feelings from behavior can be instructive in understanding a situation. But when you do surmise a person's feelings, be sure to identify it as someone's best guess, preferably someone who knows the person well. And if a person can describe how he or she is feeling, be sure to understand and use his or her own words when inferring feelings.

Environmental Events

Pay special attention to what happens before, during, and after a behavior. For example, some things in the environment can act as signals for behavior to occur. Hearing music can make us dance, smelling food can make us eat, and seeing certain people can make us smile or frown. The presence of these signals or *cues* can help us learn new ways of behaving. They can act as a "reminder" that an action needs to occur.

events before, during, and after behavior

Behavior also is influenced by what follows it. Learning and changing behavior is more easily accomplished when the consequences of a behavior are carefully determined. The consequences of a behavior can increase, decrease, or keep the rate of the behavior the same.

Context

The chain of events before, during, and after behavior does not occur in a vacuum. Look at events in the environment by considering the **context** in which things are happening for the individual. There is always a context to behavior we must try to understand. One of the most important of these is the person's established social relationships in the setting where the behavior occurs. Does the person trust and care about those around him or her? Is the person comfortable and secure? Any or all of these things can influence the way a person behaves at any moment. Some other things to explore are:

- What is important to this person?
- Why is it important?
- How does the person react and what does this tell us?
- What are the person's past experiences with this situation?
- What are his or her expectations and hopes?
- What relationships does the person have with others in this setting?
- Is the person attentive and alert?
- How does the person feel?
- Is the setting warm, cool, bright, uncomfortable?

behavior has a context

Behavior analysis is a very useful tool when trying to understand what a person is perceiving in a situation, or when assisting people to grow in their skills. For example, it can be used to plan how to best teach how to dress, shop, and communicate. Behavior analysis is also useful for understanding why certain behaviors occur, and for teaching new, more effective behavior. By carefully analyzing situations over time, we can learn much about why people act in certain ways. This, in turn, helps us to restructure situations **in partnership** with individuals so their skills and effective behavior grow.

Ways to Respond to Behavior

There are many ways for people to respond to behavior. Psychologist classify three main types of response: you can *reward* it, *ignore* it, or *punish* it. This will affect the likelihood of that action being repeated. Suppose you're driving to work and you come to a yellow traffic light. For many of us, that is a cue to step on the accelerator. But if it turns red and a police officer pulls you over for a ticket, that event likely will change, perhaps for a little while, your future behavior at yellow lights.

A behavior is rewarded when what follows it makes it more likely the behavior will occur again. When a behavior is ignored or punished, it is more likely that the rate of the behavior will decrease. There are many different ways to respond within each of these response types.

But the trouble with these basic responses is that they can oversimplify a complex situation. An even better way to think about "responding" to a behavior is to **first try to understand** it and **help the individual realize the implications the behavior has**. This might involve discussing the behavior, researching and changing the environment, modeling effective behavior, or counseling the individual.

Reinforcers

When the frequency of a behavior is maintained or increased, the consequences after that behavior are called *reinforcers*. **Reinforcers are essential for learning** because they help establish a positive approach while providing feedback to the individual about effective behaviors. Everyone uses reinforcers as a way of teaching and learning. If you handle a difficult situation with a person well and a respected colleague says, "You did a good job," you likely will use the same interpersonal approach again. If so, you were reinforced. Whether we are aware of it or not, reinforcement is important for all of us. When that colleague reinforced you, she or he helped you to learn and value a new skill.

There are many opportunities to reinforce behaviors in a dignified way. This makes a big difference for everyone. We all feel and act "better" if we are in a positive environment. Managers in the corporate world realize this, and receive extensive training in providing reinforcement to their staffs. People who are effectively reinforced grow, learn more, and are productive people.

It is important to be a reinforcing person and to know effective guidelines for reinforcement. If you know these guidelines, then you can help teach desirable behaviors and not reward behaviors that are not helpful for people. On the other hand, you must be careful not to take control of reinforcement in an effort to arbitrarily control or change the actions of people with disabilities. This is especially true of those things that people have access to as a human right.

> "The apparent simplicity of (behavioral) principles makes them more available to persons who do not completely understand them or those they use them on. This promotes bad treatment under the guise of 'science' and helps keep persons with challenges away from us..."

• *Reinforcers should be available whenever possible in the natural setting.*

If you provide reinforcers that are not normally available, the person may come to rely on those artificial rewards to function in that setting. He or she will face a difficult challenge to become more self-sufficient. Reinforcers also should not make people stand out as different. Artificial tokens or extraordinary reinforcers can make the person appear unusual to others. For example, when an adult is rewarded with "points," people in the setting may view the person as strange or different. You also should not reinforce people with childish rewards or activities.

Artificial programs may change behavior, but ultimately do very little to meet a person's real needs. These kinds of reinforcers are also difficult to leave behind when learning has occurred, creating a dependency that the regular environment cannot support. Also, as mentioned earlier, we always must ask what usefulness even an effective program serves, if in carrying it out we belittle, demean, or make someone look very different, silly, or childish.

Understanding how reinforcement works is an important tool for anyone who teaches new skills or tries to help people change ineffective behaviors. When you utilize reinforcement correctly and respectfully, you can help individuals enhance their own capabilities and self-image. When reinforcement is manipulated as a power and control tool, people usually tend to find ways to "beat the system." This is true for all of us.

• *Reinforcers must be authentic and appropriate to the context and person.*

It can be very demeaning to have your boss flatter your work in a way that you know is insincere—or for someone to reinforce an adult with a "smile sticker." Reinforcers need to be age-appropriate and real. They also should fit the setting and situation, as well as the person.

• *Reinforcers are best provided by those in the natural setting who normally provide them to others.*

Reinforcers should be not only ones that are a part of the given setting, they also should be provided whenever possible by those who are typically there. For example, rather than providing direct reinforcement to a supported employee learning a new task, a job coach should support a co-worker or supervisor to do so.

• *Reinforcers for new learning should be immediate and consistent.*

Many of us learn to delay receiving rewards for our efforts, such as working for a weekly paycheck, or even working four years for a diploma or degree. But to learn new behavior, the most effective reinforcement is immediate feedback. That way we learn clearly what exact behavior is being reinforced.

When learning a new behavior over a period of time, a person also will benefit from predictability. If reinforcement changes so that it becomes too unpredictable based on that behavior, it is not as likely to occur.

reinforcers in the natural setting

• *Reinforcer should be available in appropriate amounts.*

Sometimes people get so much of a reinforcer that it is no longer reinforcing. This is called *satiation.* Suppose you buy some new music by your favorite singer. At first you listen to it a lot. But after a while, you get tired of hearing the same song and you put something different on the stereo.

Satiation means that a reinforcer has temporarily lost its reinforcing properties. You probably will start to play your favorite music again after not listening to it for a while. The best way to avoid satiation is to be aware of and use a wide variety of effective and practical reinforcers.

- *Reinforcers are more effective when they are individualized.*

We all have differences about what things are reinforcing and how powerful each reinforcer is. We should not make assumptions about what will act as a reinforcer for people. Reinforcers vary from person to person. There are several ways to determine the best reinforcers for each individual.

Probably the easiest and best way to decide on reinforcers is to ask the person you are helping to learn. When you ask the first time, a person may have difficulty telling you. But with experience, she or he will find it easier. If a person has difficulty communicating, be a sensitive observer. Watch what the person prefers to do. It is usually easy to tell when someone enjoys something or is completely immersed in an activity. Talking honestly with a person is a very good method for choosing reinforcers. An individual always should be involved in decisions about their life and learning.

individualized reinforcement

If a given behavior increases in rate, then it is being reinforced in some way. If Mike starts making his bed much more often, he is probably being reinforced for it. Maybe someone he respects is telling him how nice his room looks when the bed is made; maybe Mike is reinforced just by seeing his own neat room. While observing, you will notice what different people prefer to do. These activities are possible reinforcers.

The guidelines for reinforcement provided here are to help you be an effective teacher, or to be a trainer of others in the community who will teach. This begins by being able to analyze behavior and help each individual understand what might be influencing his or her actions. You then should help structure settings in non-intrusive ways so that more effective and useful behavior can be learned.

Understanding your role in this process as someone who can provide support is important. Teaching tools such as reinforcement also can be abused in order to control or manipulate someone's behavior. Rather, use them as part of a technology of assistance that we all have in our lives.

Problems with Using Punishment

Another method of influencing behavior involves using punishment. The word *punishment* has a legal and a programmatic meaning. When punishment is used legally, it refers to penalties or infliction of pain or loss. **Punishment that causes physical, emotional, or psychological harm or discomfort is restricted** in programs for individuals with developmental disabilities in most states. These practices include hitting, verbal abuse, giving a cold shower, or using any technology that has the purpose of causing someone pain.

Punishment also has a programmatic meaning related to learning theory. It refers to a specific procedure in behavior analysis. Punishment is the presentation of **an unpleasant consequence that decreases the frequency of a behavior it follows.** The unpleasant consequence is called a *punisher* or an *aversive*.

The use of aversive procedures to reduce or eliminate someone's specific behavior is also restricted in most locations. Seclusion, for example, is not allowed in most states. You should review the guidelines for behavior programs with your supervisor to clarify what is restricted. These kinds of approaches to behavior change are unwarranted, not only due to violations of **personal respect for the individual**, but also because it is not as effective as a learning strategy:

> **The use of punishment can be an affront to personal dignity. People who receive punishment do not learn alternative ways to behave, the effect of suppressing the behavior can be temporary, and there are serious side effects such as avoiding the punisher or the learning environment.**

1. Punishment does not teach new appropriate behaviors.
2. Punishment is generally effective only for the time it is in use.
3. There are positive alternatives to punishment.
4. The use of punishment procedures generates detrimental side effects:
    *   **Escape/avoidance**: the person who is being punished might avoid or try to escape from the environment where the punishment occurs.
    *   **Decrease in the rate of all behavior**: the person who is being punished might begin to suppress appropriate behaviors as well as the behavior that is being punished.
    *   **Inability to deliver positive reinforcers**: the person supporting learning may be too focused trying to find and punish behavior rather than helping someone develop more effective actions.
    *   **Physiological side effects**: the use of punishment can cause muscle tension and increased respiration and blood pressure, both for the person being punished and the punisher.
    *   **Poor role model**—the person being punished might learn and imitate punishment as a means of control.

- **Learning new problem behaviors**—the person can learn new, troubling behaviors to avoid punishment. For example, an individual may begin lying to avoid punishment.

**side effects
of punishment**

Positive Alternatives to Changing Behaviors

Helping people to change ineffective behavior using principles of behavior analysis in respectful, non-aversive ways requires an investment. You need to develop an understanding of the person, creativity in the environment, a shared value system of mutual dignity, and a complete knowledge of behavior technology. A key to this will be our own actions and attitudes when interacting with the person. Whenever possible and realistic, take preventative steps that respect the person's wishes. Restructure interactions so they teach the positive results of interdependency. Some basic rules of thumb when challenging behavior interferes with this are the following:

- *Communication*:

  Observe behavior carefully and try to understand what it is telling you.

- *Personal Life Goals*

  Review the individual's interests, needs, hopes, and fears within the setting. Talk to friends, family, co-workers, and others who may provide information. Note discrepancies between what the setting offers and what the person wants or needs. Spend time with the individual and, depending on the relationship and communication capabilities, try to assess what the person wants and needs to say about his or her work.

> You need to develop an understanding of the person, creativity in the environment, a shared value system of mutual dignity, and a complete knowledge of behavior technology.

- *Observation*

  Observe the general functioning of the setting. Observe also the individual performing in the setting and talk to others about the situation. Try to determine which behavior fits acceptable norms and which does not.

- *Relationships*

  Understand the social networking in the setting and in the individual's life. Assist the person in developing friendships and other social supports.

- *Personality*

  Try to learn the unique capacities and need for support of the person based on such things as personality, performance style, learning style, history of performance, medical needs, and mobility.

- *Restructuring*

  Negotiate with the person and others to change the setting or situation so that the onset of the behavior is less likely.

- *Redirection*

  At its beginning, calmly and safely help interrupt and redirect unsafe behavior to more useful responses.

- *Reinforcement*

  Work with the person to develop situations where natural and authentic reinforcement occurs based on the occurrence of more useful behavior, and reduce the potential reinforcement of the less useful behavior.

- *Counseling*

  Seek to advise and support the person about how and why behavior change is helpful. Help the individual learn about the implications of his or her behavior.

- *Teaching and Modeling*

  Help each person gain access to social situations where positive role models are available and act as a model yourself for functional ways of behaving.

- *Documenting Learning*

  Keep good records to help guide future teaching. When people get caught up in day-to-day issues, they may lose perspective of accomplishment. Provide a larger context for people to place their daily efforts.

- *Technology*

  Apply technology to help people manage their environment and to minimize their frustration.

- *Respect*

  When your style of interaction is dignified with each person, people feel more valued and act more respectfully in return.

Safeguarding Behavioral Practices

Much of the behavior technology that has been used in the human services field to change challenging behavior consists of many techniques defined in research. These include selective use of reinforcement, redirection techniques, and other highly technical approaches. While many of these are effective, in some situations these "solutions" can be more damaging to the person and his or her reputation than the behavior itself.

One concern is that the person applying technology to change someone's actions can make decisions about which behaviors are "inappropriate" within a setting. This type of behavioral decision-making has numerous pitfalls. For one thing, it could lead to a struggle over who "controls" a given situation, the individual being assisted or the human services support person. It also can impart more decision-making over someone's life than is justified.

> There are some things in our lives that should not be manipulated, controlled, or used as a contingency. Basic human dignity and rights mean that we should never hold back our relationships with our friends to shape their responses. A friendship is given freely, and should not be contingent on unrelated behaviors which we or others are trying to change. We might get annoyed or angry at a friend's behavior, we might express our feelings, or even change our relationship, but we do not turn our relationships off or on depending on "target behaviors." Some things in life just come non-contingently, with no strings attached.

Practical use of behavior technology is a helpful change agent and skill builder for all of us. But it should be applied only with understanding and empathy and in cooperation with the individual involved and the setting he or she is in.

And there are other considerations in natural settings that must be considered before any behavioral approach is developed. For example, all of the factors mentioned earlier when analyzing behavior should be reviewed, including health; state of hunger or thirst; comfort, mood, or attentiveness; background lighting, noise, and temperature; and one's history of experiences (see C-4). Also, as we have learned, we also should consider what the person is telling us with his or her actions.

Be wary of using behavioral practices in ways that set up issues of power and control struggles. For instance, some people have used behavior programming to focus on changing someone who is labelled "non-compliant," usually defined as not conforming to directives. Without considering the person's situation, there is little thought to the context and the person's needs within it. Most everyone has been "non-compliant" when asked to do something we have no interest or desire to do. In fact, disobeying may even be a survival skill in some situations. While it is true that there are times when we must follow someone's directives, we usually have some

behavior technology is not about winning power and control

control over whether we want to be in the situation in the first place.

Even the use of reinforcement can create situations of abuse. For instance, **reinforcers should not be applied or withheld to impose control, nor should people have to earn reinforcers that are legally and ethically part of everyday life.** This is very important, as there are some things in our lives that we do that should not be manipulated, controlled, or used as a contingency. Basic human dignity and rights mean that:

- friendships shouldn't be qualified with "only if you do ..."
- meals and nutrition should not be compromised with "when you finish ..."
- privacy and personal possessions should not be removed with "since you did not..."

In our efforts to help people change behaviors and learn new ones, there is always a danger that we take on unnecessary control and authority. A few persons can present very challenging behaviors—they may do things that risk injury to others or themselves. It is our task to help each individual understand what natural consequences likely will occur, and to teach and model alternative ways of communicating, reacting to frustration, or dealing with stress.

Summary

The sensitive use of behavior principles can be an effective tool in helping an individual learn new skills and better and more useful behavior. This is crucial to successful participation in settings where the community expects certain behaviors. Whether on the job, at home, or in a store, knowing how to act and manage in the environment determines how we are perceived and what we accomplish.

But the potential for abusing this technology is great. The use of special language, the scientific aura, and the power of controlling challenging problems with oversimplified practices is alluring. Further, people with disabilities are vulnerable to how we define their "problems" and our "solutions." We must understand both the productive use of principles of behavior change and the harmful potential consequences of relegating someone to an object of a program.

Every agency is required to establish policies and procedures regarding the use of behavior principles. Review these documents along with your human rights policies before participating in the use of any behavior programs. When developing programs, remember to:

• Treat each individual with the same respect you would want for yourself.

• Act as a good model for behaviors. One of your most important teaching tools is how you act in different situations.

Some Assumptions about Respectful Behavior Practices

• It is best not to ignore dramatic bids for attention. Ignoring only encourages a person to become more dramatic. It is better voluntarily to give attention to a person sooner than be forced into giving it later.

• The way a person acts should produce as natural a result as possible. Saying to a person, "When you threaten to hurt yourself with broken glass, we will have to get you help for this problem" is a more natural consequence than saying, "If you don't stop doing this, we will punish you with restraint or medication or loss of privileges."

• When we pay attention to what a person does, we are not necessarily "reinforcing that behavior." We are opening the opportunity for a dialogue with the person. When we ask, "What does this mean for you?" we are making the first step to answering the question, "How can we help?" The second step is to say, "If you need help with something, here is another way to ask for it." This message can be trusted only if we have demonstrated that we are worthy of trust.

— Herb Lovett
Cognitive Counseling and Persons With Special Needs

POSTSESSION REVIEW

Name _____   Agency _____

Program _____   Trainer _____

Date _____   Score _____

1. In using behavior analysis, describe behavior exactly as it is:

    a. caused   b. inferred   c. deduced   d. observed

2. Some settings have expected rules for behaving. Why is it important for people to be aware of these rules?

3. In what ways can using principles to change behavior help to contribute to people's growth and learning?

4. What should be your concerns with using a behavior program that uses "smile stickers" for an adult to wear as a reinforcer for appropriate grocery shopping?

5. When a behavior is reinforced, it is likely that the behavior will _____.

6. What would be some likely ways of working with a person who speaks too loudly when she or he is in a library or bank?

7. True or False

_____ Reinforcers should be delivered immediately.

_____ Reinforcers should be delivered consistently.

_____ Quantity of reinforcement makes little difference on behavior.

_____ It's safe to assume that if one person likes something, then it would work for others as a reinforcer.

8. If you want to support a person to change an ineffective behavior that may be harmful to others, which one of the following should not be considered?

    a. an analysis of what the behavior is communicating

    b. a review of the relationships in the person's life

    c. determining how to best restrict reinforcers, such as meals

    d. an analysis of the setting and the demands and reinforcers in it

9. List at least two serious problems with using punishment.

10. In what ways can the principles of behavior analysis be misused? Use an example.

Part D

Helping People Learn Useful Skills

In previous sections of this manual, we discussed the kinds of typical social roles people with disabilities should have to be a successful community member. We also reviewed the kinds of community behavioral norms expected and some ways to help people acquire those functional behaviors.

There are also many other everyday things we all need or want to do in life. Chores at home, developing friendships, or working for an employer are examples of these. To succeed in each of these areas requires, among other things, the skills to get them done well. Learning these skills requires good teaching, the right settings and goals, and opportunities to learn and practice.

People with disabilities, including those who have difficulties with learning, are able to master very complex and meaningful skills when they receive effective training and support. In order to succeed, they may need extra assistance or some technology support. Like all of us, they will need sufficient learning opportunities, enough time to learn, and the right amount of practice not to forget.

> Deciding what to teach, where to teach, who will teach, and how to teach are some of the most important decisions you will make with the persons you will support. The purpose of teaching is to assist people with disabilities to live, work, and play in the community settings of their choice.

For these reasons, the approach you use to help people learn skills is very important. Deciding with someone what to learn, where learning will occur, who will teach, and how things will be taught are some of the most important decisions you will make. The purpose of any of your teaching is to assist people to live, work, and recreate successfully in the community settings of their choice.

There are many important things to remember about teaching and learning. One of the most vital is to view teaching as a partnership. A two-way street exists between a teacher and the learner in a particular setting. You should not approach a learning situation to control or manipulate someone's life, but to work together as equals to support new ways of doing things.

Individual Service Plan

Writing an *Individual Service Plan* (ISP) is also part of the teaching process. A service plan such as an ISP is required in every state where public funding is used to provide needed services for people with disabilities. This plan should make clear the supports and strategies needed and desired by an individual to significantly improve his or her quality of life. The plan should be a flexible guide based on what decisions the person expresses, along with the input of family, friends, and other advocates and people in the person's life.

This section provides an overview of planning teaching strategies to help a person learn the skills he or she needs and wants for a better lifestyle.

Determining What to Learn

- **The person should direct the assessment of what areas to develop and enhance.**

Deciding what things a person should learn should be based on the future goals and lifestyle the person wishes to pursue. There are numerous ways to determine this. The individual and his or her ISP can help tell you what he or she enjoys, wishes to learn, and can already do. The combination of what the person can do and his or her hopes, desires, skills, and interests leads to the development of an individual support plan. Based on this and other information, you and the person can make good choices about what to teach, what to adapt, or when to assist.

> A thoughtful staff person who helps a person decide on teaching goals and strategies will need to use good judgement. Avoid spending too much time teaching difficult skills you think a person must master before he or she is "ready" for a job, his or her own home, or a community activity.

For example, Joan has just decided to move into a home in a new community. She wants to work nearby and to be able to get to her job on her own. She does not know many safety rules, but she wants to learn to walk to a job she has been offered. It would be useful for her to choose your assistance from among the following options:

- Help her learn how to walk safely to work.
- Help her find someone to walk with her to work.
- Provide her assistance in arranging her own ride.
- Help her arrange her work schedule to make it easier for her to reach her goal.

Rather than just picking the most convenient solution, discuss with Joan what new skills and behaviors would be best to learn now, and what things in the environment should be changed for her to reach her goal. Since this is such an individualized process, learning should occur **one person at a time**. Training activities for groups of people with disabilities tend to limit the capabilities of each person, and also produces the negative labeling effects discussed in Part B.

> People who have disabilities are at particular risk of spending their entire lives in preparatory training. Some persons never experience a full community life because of someone's arbitrary judgement that they are not ready.

- **Some situations are better approached by providing help or modifications.**

Struggling for a long time to learn a skill that is difficult to master can delay an important life goal for too long. When someone wants to have more control over their finances, it might take too long for them to have mastery over budgeting and balancing a checkbook. Instead, they might benefit immediately from some environmental support, such as having prepaid accounts with some local stores, while they continue to work on budgeting. This is a decision that must be made carefully by the person and his or her family and service team.

Other times it may make sense for someone to learn only part of a complex task rather than the whole thing. The concept that anyone is capable of learning some part of any task is called *partial participation*. It is important because it provides opportunities for persons to contribute and participate in community settings, even though they may not easily be able to do all parts of a task.

partial participation

- **Help people learn skills that are functional.**

Functional skills involve those tasks that are done every day at home, at work, and in community settings. If an individual is unable to do these tasks, then someone probably will have to do them for him or her. This is a good yardstick to tell if the skill is important to teach.

Often in the past, teachers and trainers focused far too much effort on "readiness" skills. As a result, many persons with disabilities spent all their time with pre-vocational training, or practicing skills in a classroom instead of participating and learning in the community. Learning everyday functional skills in the setting where they are to be used is a far more useful way to spend valuable time.

- **Support learning skills that are age-appropriate.**

As mentioned earlier, persons with disabilities are subject to many myths. One of these is being seen as childlike, or as "never growing up." In order to promote dignity and change this harmful myth, work with the person on skills for adulthood. The learning materials should be those things with which most adults would be

age appropriateness

comfortable. This means not using pegboards, blocks, beads, or childish puzzles and games.

Before choosing and defining what to teach, ask the following questions:

- Is it age appropriate?
- Is it functional?
- Is it a personal preference?
- Is it a family/guardian preference?
- Does it help improve reputation?
- Does it help promote positive relationships?
- Is it likely to be learned?

Many people with developmental disabilities **learn best when taught precisely**. Therefore, you should define exactly what needs to be taught. It is best not to leave learning to chance. Earlier sections explain how to define and observe behavior. Based on this information, you can decide on useful and realistic learning goals and objectives.

Determining Where to Learn

competent models

- **A person learns best in the presence of competent models.**

When a person receives instruction, one person at a time, in a setting where the people around him or her are competent, that person is seen as a productive individual and is less defined by his her disability label. People can imitate useful, effective behavior only when they are learning with capable models.

natural environments

- **A person learns best in the setting where the skill is required.**

Although people with developmental disabilities can successfully learn many types of complex skills, many individuals do not **generalize** these skills very well. This means that they have difficulty transferring what they learn from one environment to another. It is more effective, then, to start teaching in the environment where the person will need to perform, rather than spending needless time "getting ready" before attempting to learn community activities and work.

- **A person learns best in real situations and with real materials, rather than artificial ones.**

When we try to simulate an environment, we leave out many important variables. This can interfere with learning later in the "real" situation. Use materials and settings the person will need to perform the skill.

For example, many programs utilize "simulated work" for vocational readiness training. This work often bears little resemblance to any community job that a person would like to have, and it rarely helps the individual in his or her performance on a job site. Even when simulated work is related to a particular job, it is far more effective and useful to support a person in the actual setting doing real work.

• **A person learns best when using learning opportunities within the natural setting where the skill is to be used.**

natural supports

These types of learning exchanges that are a typical part of a setting are known as *natural supports*. This is the kind of support that members of a community provide to each other. Not only is encouraging natural supports an effective training strategy, it also helps a person belong socially in the fabric of a community. One of the greatest difficulties disability professionals face is the seeming dependency people with disabilities have on our presence and support. But this is more often due to our view of our role as the primary source of all teaching and caretaking for the person.

Determining Who Will Support Learning

While there may be many situations where human services professionals indeed need to provide teaching, there are many others where **the people in community settings can help teach the rules and skills expected there**. One advantage to this approach is that the training comes from those who best know the task to be learned.

A good example is in supported employment. Learning a job can often result from the instruction of co-workers and supervisors. This same approach can occur in other settings. The bank teller, for instance, can offer assistance on personal checking. Family and friends also may be a source of training support for other areas of community life. Our role, then, is to be a consultant and resource to help make sure needed learning occurs in the most effective way.

Summary of Key Learning Principles

1. Assess with the person, areas to develop and enhance.
2. Define with the individual what to teach.
3. Help the person learn skills and behaviors based on his or her individual wants and needs.
4. Use teaching strategies that match the strengths among the multiple intelligences of the person.
5. Assist the person to learn functional skills.
6. Help the person learn in age-appropriate ways.
7. Teach in the setting where the skill is required.
8. Use real situations and materials, rather than artificial ones.
9. Facilitate natural learning opportunities.

Determining How to Learn

- **Determine the most effective way to approach the task to be learned.**

When a skill to be learned requires a sequence of behaviors, it can be difficult to master. A solution to helping someone learn a complex skill is to break the set of behaviors down into steps. For example, learning to operate a dishwasher consists of many different operations that generally should proceed in a certain order. By breaking these steps down into small learning bits, an individual can concentrate on one step at a time, such as measuring detergent.

teachable steps

A *task analysis* organizes an activity to be learned into *teachable steps* and strategies for instruction. It allows the learner to develop multistep, complex skills that otherwise would be difficult to acquire. Each individual will set her or his own content for what is a teachable step. John may need to focus only on pouring the detergent, while Ray may be able to learn to get out the detergent, pour it, close the door, and turn on the machine at one time.

The first step in developing a task analysis is to decide on a method of performing the activity. There are usually many ways to do any task. Most people have their own unique way of putting on their jacket, for instance. Choosing the method depends on many factors, which should lead to the best available alternative. Always consider **the most natural way** of doing a task for the learner, as well as **the most accepted method** in the setting it is to be performed.

> A task analysis should utilize the most natural way of doing a task for the learner and the setting.

Once a method is selected, develop a list of the teachable steps in the order they normally occur. Once this is accomplished, decide on instructional strategies such as setting, materials, order of teaching the steps, reinforcement, length of learning sessions, and natural cues. Here is a simple example of a task analysis for dialing a telephone, using a cue card with a telephone number.

1. *Grasp handle of phone receiver.*
2. *Lift receiver to above shoulder.*
3. *Place listening part of receiver to ear.*
4. *Pause for two seconds; listen for dial tone.*
5. *Using the other hand, touch the first number to be dialed on the card and say it aloud.*
6. *Move your finger to the matching number printed on one of the phone push-buttons.*
7. *Press the button for the number.*
8. *Remove your finger from the button.*
9. *Repeat steps 6 to 8 for each number.*
10. *Pause and listen for phone to ring.*

• **Determine the most effective learning style for the person.**

In 1983 Howard Gardner wrote a book entitled *Frames of Mind: The Theory of Multiple Intelligences*. According to Gardner, there is not a single intelligence, as measured by one IQ score. Instead, there are different kinds of intelligences, giving people a new way to think about learning. He defined seven different kinds of intelligence, noting that people will vary in abilities across all these dimensions. The seven areas are:

• Linguistic: a sensitivity to the meaning and order of words
• Logical-mathematical
• Musical
• Spatial: the ability to "think in pictures"
• Bodily-kinesthetic: the ability to use one's body in a skilled way, for self-expression or toward a goal
• Interpersonal: an ability to perceive and understand other individuals
• Intrapersonal: an understanding of one's own emotions

Recently, Gardner has identified an eighth intelligence, naturalistic, or the ability to recognize and classify plants, minerals, and animals.

This theory means that the reason some people have learning problems is because they might not be having an opportunity to excel using their particular gifts. Of course, we still must be very careful about using these intelligences as labels of any kind, but trainers need to consider very seriously individual differences among the people they teach. A trainer must look at what each person could do well, instead of what he or she cannot do.

Instruction also should support the natural intelligence each person has. If someone is linguistic, then you should use language to explain something. But if someone is more intelligent spatially, then using pictures as cues might be better. Or if someone is more skilled in bodily movement, helping them physically learn a routine through guidance might be more beneficial.

For example, Jim learns best when you show him what to do so that he can imitate you. When Jim begins to learn how to cut his food when eating, arrange for him to watch someone cut his or her food, then encourage him to imitate. If Jim is learning how to file at work, encourage his co-worker to demonstrate filing rather than try to verbally explain it to him.

Each person learns best in certain ways. When teaching a new skill, use the style that the person prefers.

multiple intelligences

learning styles

> Be aware of disability images and myths so teaching experiences do not make people look different, childish, or unusual. This includes knowing how, what, when, and most importantly, why we support learning.

Giving Assistance during Learning

There are a variety of teaching supports available to help the learner. For example, when you teach new behaviors, you can use helpful *prompts*. Prompts are brief instructional *cues* or signals given before the response to help the person when learning something new.

There are three main types of prompts to teach skills:

prompts

- *Auditory* prompts: verbal instructions or hints
- *Visual* prompts: pictures, gestures, or demonstrations
- *Tactile* prompts or physical guidance prompts: touching or guiding through a skill

Here are general guidelines to consider when using prompts to teach new behaviors:

natural cues

1. Determine and **use prompts that are a natural part of the setting**. For example, a laundry buzzer, a full hamper of laundry, a cooking timer, or a scheduled work break each can signal something to be done. There can be a variety of other signals from equipment, schedules, clocks, people, and other parts of the environment where the person is to use the skill. These *natural cues* should be used as much as possible in all learning situations.

minimal necessary assistance

2. In order for learning to take place, a person needs an adequate opportunity to attempt the task. For this to occur, you should provide only the **least assistance needed for the person to succeed.**

3. Use consistent, descriptive vocal prompts. **Reduce extra words in directions.** If the least-needed vocal prompt can be nonspecific ("what's next?"), use that rather than giving a direction.

4. Use an unexcited tone of voice for a vocal prompt. When you reinforce a behavior, use a naturally expressive voice. This helps to **distinguish a prompt from other verbal behavior**, including reinforcement.

> Always begin with the most natural assistance possible. Prompts should fit the conditions of the setting, taking into consideration norms, safety, and comfort. The personal preferences and learning style of the individual also need to be understood.

5. Give a vocal or a visual prompt before giving a guidance prompt. This will **provide an opportunity for the person to initiate the desired behavior** him or herself. People can become dependent more easily on physical guidance.

6. **Support self-instruction**. Recent research has demonstrated the power of teaching people to *self-instruct*. This is a training strategy that helps individuals to better master learning more indepen-

dently. The person first observes a competent task performer who successfully completes the task while speaking the instructions out loud. The person then performs the task while the trainer continues to instruct, and eventually performs the task while self-instructing aloud.

> **The most effective use of reinforcement to enhance learning is to use non-artificial, naturally occurring reinforcers that are available to everyone who participates in the learning setting.**

Reinforcing Learning

Another tool for enhancing learning is to use the principles of reinforcement as discussed in Part C. As a person learns to perform a behavior more fluidly and accurately with the prompts one provides, the trainer should reinforce that behavior to make it more likely to reoccur. There are generally many natural reinforcers available for learning, including the self-satisfaction of mastering a new skill, increased wages on a job, or the social praise of those the person cares about.

reinforcement natural to the setting and the skill

Reinforcement works best when it is provided immediately, when it is contingent on the performance, and when it is consistent, authentic, and truly reinforcing. Reinforcers should be appropriate to the age and setting, and should occur naturally within the setting and task. The schedule for reinforcers should move from intensive and continuous to a more natural and sporadic level as the person masters more of the skill.

Using reinforcement as a tool for learning can be very effective. But you must remember that inserting artificial or unusual types of reinforcement can damage the learner's reputation and status. If you become too rigid with reinforcement, you also have too much control over a person's life.

Assisting to Avoid or Correct Errors

During the course of learning, an individual will probably make mistakes. A good teacher anticipates likely mistakes. You then can choose when best to provide needed assistance. This requires good judgement. You must allow for challenge, risk, and growth within a learning opportunity. You also must try to minimize frustration and incorrect behaviors that may interfere with effective learning.

When a learner has made a mistake, it is usually best to gently interrupt immediately in order to repeat the step correctly. Again, provide the least amount of assistance necessary. A natural environmental interruption is preferable. You should be sensitive to the setting and the person, and try not to be intrusive.

Remember to be aware of the learning potential of modeling. There is a powerful relationship between your own behavior and the person you teach.

Sometimes the behavior of correcting an individual acts as a reinforcer because of the interaction that occurs. When your assistance is actually interfering with learning, it is best to consider alternative strategies for learning with the person. One idea is to develop ways for the individual to be able to review his or her own work and make self-corrections.

Fading Learning Assistance

The advantage of using prompts in teaching is that they help to initiate new, desirable behavior. A possible disadvantage is that some people become too dependent on prompts that are not a natural part of the setting to complete the task. This disadvantage can be solved by *fading* the prompts as soon as possible. Fading is an important part of the teaching process because it helps a person to work and function with less artificial supports.

Fading to More Natural Reinforcement

Fading the level of reinforcers provided during instruction will encourage a more natural, uninterrupted performance of the task. As the person becomes more proficient, the quantity of reinforcers should be reduced, while the number of steps needed to reach reinforcement should increase. Ultimately, the person should be able to perform the skill based on the natural reinforcement available from the setting or the internal satisfaction of accomplishment. Again, this should be a gradual process to build performance, not create frustration.

Fading Prompts

One way to fade is by using a slightly smaller, less guided cue each time the person performs the task. For example, you may have helped someone learn how to locate cereal by using verbal prompts. You could begin fading by reducing these prompts and using simpler instructions, then a nonspecific instruction ("where do you look first?"), then, if necessary, only a pointing cue or a small picture card on the cabinet until it is no longer necessary.

Developing Natural Support

Another part of the process of fading is to build bridges of support to the natural environment for each area where someone might need assistance. The best way to reduce trainer dependency is to be sure that the setting provides any needed cues. Environments often have all sorts of possible signals and reminders built into them. Fade from prompts that are not a part of the natural environment, and direct the learner to the natural cues of the setting.

Building Generalization

Still another facet of fading is to help the learner generalize newly learned skills so he or she can use them in a variety of situations and settings. Once someone has mastered a skill in one setting, for example, you should choose new settings where he or she can continually experience success. This process also can be done with different materials, times, or situations so the person can perform the skill in many circumstances.

Fading is thus an active process and does not mean arbitrarily reducing your presence. Whenever possible, you are looking for support and learning experiences that can become "self-sustaining," rather than dependent on outside assistance. The reduction of your time spent supporting someone in a community setting is not the process of fading, it is the outcome. If you succeed in building natural supports over time, and if the person generalizes the skills he or she needs to use, your presence becomes less and less needed. Needed supports also evolve and change, of course. Providing ongoing, flexible support to the person and the community environment is a part of being a good teacher.

self-sustaining skills

Using Good Teaching Practices

Whether you have developed a teaching relationship between a person with a disability and someone in the community, or you are providing the teaching yourself, you will need to demonstrate effective teaching strategies. Some guidelines follow:

• **Be consistent when you teach.**

Consistency is particularly important when teaching a new skill. It enables people to know what to expect so they can pay attention to the task rather than to something else. Consistency can apply to the teaching area, the materials you use, the instructions you give, and the response.

• **Provide frequent and varied practice.**

People learn best when they practice something until it is mastered. But when you provide many opportunities for practice, teaching can get boring. To avoid boredom, vary your strategies. You still can be consistent while using interesting approaches.

> Ultimately, it is the teaching relationship between the learner and trainer that will ensure the success of the training.

A support person must always balance the availability of powerful instructional techniques with the needs and realities of the person and the setting.

data collection

• **Use short, frequent teaching sessions.**

It is much better to teach a skill every day for fifteen minutes rather than once a week for two hours. For example, if you are assisting someone with her or his hygiene, it would be preferable to work on a skill like tooth brushing for a few minutes every morning instead of once for a half hour every Sunday.

• **Chart progress.**

Keep a record of the teaching activity and date; the amount of supervision, help, and time needed; accuracy; accomplishments; and difficulties. This will help you plan for the next teaching opportunity. Most programs have forms and systems to keep track of learning strategies, prompting, and performance. The purpose of keeping this data is not to fill up files, but to make decisions with the person about how to best learn skills.

• **Give your full attention.**

Teaching requires a full-time effort.

• **Act as a good model.**

The language and behavior that you present is often what individuals will learn.

• **At appropriate times, talk about the activity you are doing.**

It is easy to forget to do this, especially when you are around someone who doesn't speak.

• **Treat each person with respect.**

Don't talk about the people with whom you work as if they weren't there.

• **Use your body language for communication.**

Your voice, body position, posture, mood, and facial expression will express information the learner can use.

• **Seek out indications and confirmation of learning.**

Don't automatically assume that a person either understands or doesn't understand what you are saying. Each person has different levels of comprehension.

Summary

Your role is to provide meaningful opportunities for persons with disabilities to participate in a community as workers, neighbors, and friends. This makes it crucial to facilitate the learning of skills in an enhancing way.

You need to be skilled at helping people in their choices about what to learn, when to learn, how to learn, and why to learn. You should be skilled in assessing strengths, learning styles, and difficulties. Be aware of images and myths so your teaching does not make people look different, childish, or unusual. Understand teaching and its process—prompting, reinforcing, fading, and other techniques. For individuals with disabilities, like all of us, **time is valuable. We should spend it wisely, creatively, and effectively as enhancers of life experiences, facilitators of social relationships, and teachers of functional skills.**

Skills on the Job

"It's great having Pat here...we really enjoy having her as an employee," summed up Neil Johnson, manager of Eastern Mountain Sports. "Pat" is Pat Park, who is responsible for keeping the merchandise in the vast EMS sales floor neat and orderly.

"Pat has really developed into a valued employee," said Johnson. "At first, she had a short attention span. Now she has developed the ability to stay with something."

Johnson has also seen Park begin to join in as part of the close-knit EMS staff. "At the start, Pat was introverted and not overly social," he said. "In the time she's worked here, that has changed dramatically. Now she talks with virtually all my staff at some point. She has come a long way and so have we in learning to understand her when she expresses herself."

Park, who spent much of her life in an institution for persons with developmental disabilities, has purchased a unit in a downtown housing cooperative with two other women. Her home is conveniently located to her job.

– Dawn Langton
Granite State Employment News

POSTSESSION REVIEW

Name _____   Agency _____

Program _____   Trainer_____

Date _____   Score _____

l. When a person needs help to participate in the community, a teacher should consider:
   a. modifying the environment   c. teaching a new skill
   b. providing assistance   d. all of the above

2. People with disabilities do not always transfer what they learn very well from one setting to another. This is called a difficulty with _____. With this in mind, how should you help someone learn how to use money?

3. What is a good way to assess if a skill is a functional one?

4. It's a good idea to use materials or lessons from any age level that the person you teach needs.
   True or False. Explain your answer.

5. John's teacher decides to teach shopping skills in a supermarket while shopping. Is this a good idea? _____. Why or why not?

6. Which is better for teaching a person with a learning disability:
   a. short, fifteen-minute teaching sessions every day
   b. longer, two-hour sessions once a week
   Explain your choice.

7. Name at least two things you should record when charting learning progress. Why should we keep track of learning?

8. Name three types of prompts you can use to teach behaviors.

9. Once a person has mastered a skill using a certain prompt, what techniques would you use so the person isn't dependent on the prompt? Describe.

10. Using group lessons to teach can work providing there are good role _____ in the group. Why is this necessary? What are the risks of teaching in groups?

Part E

Everyday Health and Safety

For some people with whom you work, living and working in the community might be a new experience. These individuals might need your support and guidance to maintain good personal health and safety.

Good health practices are crucial so that individuals will feel well and be able to enjoy the fullness of life. The way individuals feel and how they present themselves have a strong effect on their ability to develop friendships, succeed on a job, or simply to enjoy living. Personal health is strongly related to good hygiene, nutrition, exercise, and safety.

There are many things we can do each day that help us to be healthy. These include getting enough sleep, eating well, exercising regularly, and not smoking. The following practices are general health principles that apply to all of us. Put them to use when supporting people with disabilities.

> Good health practices are crucial for individuals to feel well and be able to enjoy the fullness of life. Personal health is strongly related to proper hygiene, nutrition, exercise, and safety.

Nutrition

Nutrition involves the food we eat and the way our bodies use this food. Different foods contain different nutrients. Each person needs certain amounts of different nutrients to maintain his or her health. Therefore, we need to eat a variety of foods each day. There are certain principles to keep in mind when planning a daily diet:

- Each of the nutrients is extremely important for different body functions.
- No food, by itself, has all the nutrients we need. For example, there are vitamins in vegetables that are not present in grains.
- An overabundance of one nutrient does not make up for the lack of another. Eating a double portion of potatoes will not make up for not eating carrots.
- To be the most effective, most nutrients need to be combined with others. If you are missing one nutrient in your diet, most of the body functions can be affected.

food groups

Foods have been classified into groups based on nutrients. Each day an adult should have a variety of foods from each, with most of our choices from the first three groups and very little of the sixth group. These groups are:

- bread, cereal, rice, pasta, and other grains, preferably whole
- vegetables
- fruits
- meat, poultry, eggs, dry beans, fish, nuts
- milk and other dairy products
- fat, oil, and sweets

People tend to ignore eating fruits and vegetables most often, yet there are many vitamins and minerals found only in this food group. For adults, the challenge is to eat servings from each group and not gain extra weight. In most cases, avoiding sweets and fats helps. Desserts, soda, and candy are very high in calories and provide little of the nutrients that our bodies require.

Encourage and help educate the people you support to establish a healthy diet in the following ways:

- **Avoid highly-processed foods.** Many prepackaged foods are low in nutrients and high in salt. When possible, meals should be made from fresh ingredients.

- **Choose low-fat versions of items.** Many dairy and other products are available with lower fat contents. Most labels now also list the number of grams of fat per serving.

- **Avoid sweet desserts and sugary cereals.** The contents on labels are listed in order of quantity, so it is fairly easy to find out which foods are low in sugar, corn syrup, or other types of sugars.

- **Have fresh fruit available.** It is a quick, easy snack and an excellent dessert.

- **Make vegetables appetizing.** Steam for a short period and add various herbs for seasoning, low-sodium soy sauce, or chicken broth, or a **small** amount of butter or margarine. Salads are another appetizing way to present vegetables. Try preparing with a light oil and vinegar dressing or a small amount of lemon juice.

Exercise and nutrition often are overlooked when considering the health and well-being of an individual. Yet we largely can control the food we eat and the way in which we keep active. These simple decisions can greatly influence our mental attitude and our physical health.

- **Plan menus before you shop.** Make sure you buy foods that provide daily variety in the correct proportions.

Exercise

Exercise is a very important part of good health. With the conveniences in today's lifestyles, many people don't regularly "work out." For many people, exercise helps with problems of weight control, constipation, general attitude, and many other health issues. Regular exercise helps not only physical health but emotional health as well.

It is best to exercise several times a week for fifteen to twenty minutes rather than once a week for two hours. Encourage the people you support to **build exercise into their everyday lives.** To be certain about any medical restrictions of people with whom you work, ask them to consult with their physicians before they begin a new exercise program.

> **Fitness also is strongly tied to self-image. Psychologists have learned that the way people perceive themselves is more powerful in determining personality and behavior than the way they actually look.**

Hygiene

Hygiene is an important part of health maintenance. It involves cleanliness and sanitation. Cleanliness is an extremely important factor in preventing germs from spreading and causing illness and infection.

- People should take frequent, thorough showers or baths with soap. Hair should be washed regularly, and fingernails and toenails should be trimmed and free from dirt. Clothing should be washed routinely. People should brush and floss their teeth each day.

- People should regularly use clean bed linen and clean towels. It is very important that each person uses his or her own towel since germs can easily remain and grow on wet towels. Used menstrual pads or tampons should be wrapped and thrown away in closed containers.

- Individuals should wash their hands with soap, particularly after using the bathroom.

- Homes and places of work should be clean, particularly bathrooms and kitchens. In the kitchen, the following rules should be followed:

- Wash hands and arms with soap and hot water before and after cooking and serving food, going to the toilet, and blowing your nose.
- Keep your hair tied back.
- Don't cough or sneeze near food or dishes.
- Keep food covered until it is served.
- Throw away all leftover food from someone's plate.
- Store perishable food such as milk and butter in the refrigerator at all times.
- Keep animals away from cooking surfaces.
- Keep the sink, counters, and floors very clean.

- Cover garbage and remove it frequently.

- Earaches and sore throats come from germs that enter the nose and mouth. To stop these from spreading, individuals should cover their noses and mouths with a tissue when sneezing or coughing. Throw away all dirty tissues and napkins in covered wastebaskets.

- Stomachaches and diarrhea also are usually caused by the germs on things we put in our mouths: food (contaminated by flies), dirty utensils, pencils, and fingers, for instance. You can help to prevent this by making sure food is prepared, handled, and served under the cleanliest possible conditions. Be especially sure to protect food from flies.

- Athlete's foot, impetigo, and other skin infections are caused by germs. Scabies, body lice, and other parasites also live on the skin and cause infections. They may be spread by insects or by contact with personal items such as clothing, sheets, towels, combs, and soap. You can help to control the spread of these skin infections by keeping insects out of living and working areas, and by storing the infected person's personal items separately. Clean the infected person's clothes, sheets, towels, and other washables separately.

Medical Care
Prevention

There are many things to do that help prevent medical emergencies. Here are a few:

- **Maintain a daily, healthy routine.**

- **Be safety-conscious.** Work areas should be designed with safety in mind. For example, a fire extinguisher should be near the stove.

- **Take drugs and medications only as prescribed.** Some drugs are more effective when combined with regular, healthy meals and adequate sleep. For instance, diabetes is controlled with insulin and food intake; someone with epilepsy is more likely to have a seizure if she or he has not had enough sleep.

- **Develop a working knowledge of the medications** used by the individuals with whom you work. This means understanding what the medication is and why it is prescribed. Know the dosage, frequency, and method of taking the medication; the prescribing physician; the start and end dates; storage and inventory; possible side effects; and any special considerations.

- Support individuals in **maintaining periodic health checkups.** This should include visiting their physicians, dentists, and possibly eye doctors regularly. Some people may need sensitive assistance to help with exams or health care because of difficult past experiences.

- **Maintain good health records.** Many organizations have specific ways of keeping records on medical and safety events. Learn them well for everyone's benefit.

Emergencies

Anyone can develop a serious medical condition. Some people with developmental disabilities also may have particular medical concerns. Some disabilities are associated with heart malformations or liver, pancreas, or kidney dysfunctions. Because of these kinds of problems, you may have to respond to a medical emergency. Also, some people may not be verbal or may have very limited expressive skills. Therefore, you must be able to assess symptoms to decide on the best response. For example, if a person has signs of a fever (listlessness, red cheeks, and glassy eyes), then you should take the person's temperature.

A Working Knowledge of Medications

- Understand what the medication is and why it is prescribed.
- Know the dosage, frequency, and method of taking the medication.
- Know who the prescribing physician is.
- Know the start and end dates.
- Be familiar with proper storage and inventory.
- Be aware of any special considerations for the person.
- Be responsible in taking medications only as prescribed.
- Know that some drugs are more effective when combined with regular, healthy meals and adequate sleep.
- Be aware of the possible side effects of each medication.

The first rule in an emergency is to **stay calm**. It is much easier to do this if you are prepared. **The best preparation is for all staff to have a knowledge of first-aid.** There are many courses available in first-aid sponsored by groups such as the YMCA and American Red Cross. In addition to taking a course, have a first-aid book available.

Know each person's records for her or his medical history. All staff should be aware of any medical problems. If someone has any serious medical problems and is not verbal, he or she should wear a Medic-Alert® necklace or bracelet. Maintain emergency medical information on cards that can be kept handy and transportable.

Keep emergency telephone numbers next to the phone. These should include: names of personal doctors, poison control center, hospital emergency room, rescue squad, and fire and police departments. **Have a first-aid kit on hand** at all times.

> • The best preparation is to have a knowledge of first-aid.
> • Know each person's medical history.
> • Keep emergency telephone numbers next to the phone.
> • Have a first-aid kit on hand at all times.

Mental Health

Mental health is an important part of general health. Overall, one in ten Americans experience some disability from a diagnosable mental illness in any given year. Mental illness still is largely misunderstood, feared, and stigmatized. The most severe mental illnesses include schizophrenia, manic-depressive illness, major depression, panic disorder, and obsessive-compulsive disorder.

Mental illnesses are complex disorders involving our capacities to think, feel, and act. Research has led to major advances in therapies and prevention. You should **encourage individuals to seek treatment when they find themselves experiencing the signs and symptoms of mental distress.** There are safe and effective medications and psychosocial services, typically used in combination, to effectively treat most mental disorders.

Epilepsy and Seizures

There are many different types of seizures. It is important to know if individuals have seizures and what kind they have. The three most common types of seizures are grand mal, petit mal, and psychomotor seizures.

stages of a grand mal seizure

Grand Mal

Grand mal seizures affect the whole body. They consist of the following stages:

1. **Aura:** The person may feel cold or smell something bad. These sensations are often a signal prior to the onset of the seizure.
2. **Tonic phase:** Next, a generalized contraction of the whole body likely will cause the person to cry out and/or then fall. She or he does not feel pain at this time. The jaw clamps shut and salivation increases and collects in the mouth and throat. Breathing may be interrupted and the person may turn blue. This phase usually lasts twenty to thirty seconds.
3. **Clonic phase:** In the next phase, the muscles of the body alternate with contractions and relaxations. This causes the body to twitch and jerk. The person may lose control of his or her bladder or bowel.
4. **Recovery phase:** Finally, the muscles relax. At first, the person is not arousable and may seem confused. But gradually, the person returns to an alert state.
5. **Sleepiness:** Generally, a person is very sleepy after a grand mal seizure and often has a headache.

Petit Mal

Petit mal seizures last from five to thirty seconds. They usually cause a brief loss of consciousness. The person appears to have a lapse of attention or a moment of daydreaming. Sometimes a person's face may twitch or his or her head may drop. Falling down does not usually occur. The individual will not remember the seizure. Since the symptoms are so brief, people often misinterpret or do not notice these kinds of seizures.

Psychomotor

Psychomotor seizures are very different from grand mal or petit mal seizures. A person having this kind of seizure carries on activities without being fully conscious although they may appear to be. Often, the activities are normal but done in the wrong places. For example, a person might clap his or her hands repetitively while working. Sometimes, a person may appear to be hallucinating.

Observing a seizure can be alarming. If a person has a grand mal seizure, the main rule is to **keep calm**. Remember that there is nothing you can do to stop a seizure once it has started, but there are things you can do to help:

1. **Protect the person from getting hurt**. Do not try to hold the person down, but clear the immediate area.
2. **Turn the head to the side**. If you can turn the head **without too much strain**, it will allow saliva to drain out of the mouth. Do

this only if you can do it gently. Do not try to open the mouth or put anything in the mouth. A person is unlikely to swallow his or her tongue.

3. **Do not try to interfere or stop the seizure.**

4. **Provide support after the seizure.** After a seizure, a person is usually tired and may need to rest. While recovering from a seizure, a person may have difficulty eating or drinking, so it is best not to provide food or drink until he or she fully recovers. Reassurance, a quiet word, respect, comfort, and a chance to sleep are the best things to provide.

There are some situations that call for swift medical attention. **Call a doctor or an ambulance immediately if a seizure lasts for more than three to five minutes, if a person has a series of grand mal seizures, or if the person has continued difficulty breathing.** Observing a person during a seizure is important. Reporting can help in treating seizures. The following should be noted:

1. time the seizure begins and stops
2. how it begins and body parts affected
3. anything unusual before the seizure started
4. what happened during the seizure
5. what happened after the seizure

> Call a doctor or an ambulance immediately if a seizure lasts for more than three to five minutes, if a person has continued difficulty breathing, or has a series of grand mal seizures.

anti-convulsants

Medications for Seizures

Eighty-five percent of all seizures can be controlled with *anticonvulsant* medications. It is often necessary for a person with seizures to take anti-convulsants for his or her entire life. Based on the type of seizure, a doctor may prescribe a combination of medications. Depending on the doctor's orders, a person who takes anti-convulsants may have blood drawn occasionally to monitor the amount of medication in the body.

Dental Care

Everyone wishes to keep their teeth, yet the loss of a tooth is a common occurrence. Gum disease is the major cause, and this is preventable. It is caused by plaque, a sticky buildup on teeth that should be removed. Removal takes only a few minutes a day, but it must be done properly and regularly to be effective. People should brush with a soft-bristled brush and clean between the teeth with dental floss. Learning to do this can be difficult at first for some people with physical or learning disabilities, but individuals can become proficient with support.

Even with proper brushing and flossing, some of the plaque hardens. This has to be removed professionally. Help support the people with whom you work to see their dentists regularly.

Fire Safety

Recent studies show that home fires are the largest threat to life and safety in the country. The people with disabilities you support at home and at work require your best efforts to ensure their safety from fire.

Often, evacuation from fire can be hindered by a person's mobility, ability to decide on an action, or a sensory difficulty such as blindness or deafness. Also, some individuals may have a low tolerance to smoke, particularly elderly people. Some people, including human services staff, might insist on dressing, resisting, or working to fight the fire. Resistance to evacuation is dangerous. Knowledge of the people you are with and their likely difficulties can help you anticipate evacuation problems.

Causes and Prevention

One of the ways to prevent fire is to recognize and control things that start fires:

Smoking

Help educate the individuals with whom you work, with respect and without pressure, to make an informed decision about smoking. If a person chooses to smoke, help him or her learn where doing so is permitted legally, and where it will be safe for the environment and not cause discomfort to others. Most workplaces or public settings have smoking restrictions, and you may need to explain them to anyone unclear of the rules. Provide large, deep ashtrays for tables. Do not place them on the arms of chairs. Empty ashtrays often into metal cans and keep them until cool.

Electrical

Help people to use only UL-approved appliances and regularly check for frayed or worn plugs. Remind people to keep appliances away from drapes and unplugged when not in use. Be sure exterior cords are not run under rugs. Do not delay repairs to wiring or heating systems.

> One of your responsibilities in preventing loss of life in a fire is to be familiar with each person's individual mobility needs and safety plans to evacuate.

Household

Assist people to keep the area around a furnace free from paper, paint, and wood. Keep portable heaters away from curtains, clothes, bedding, and water. Throw out rubbish regularly in metal containers. Keep cleaning materials safely stored. Do not store things in exit ways. Be especially careful when using the stove. People should keep the fire department number near the telephone.

Inspection

Maintain ongoing inspection practices as required in your local community, program, or state certification standards. This requires a working knowledge of life safety codes, state and local fire marshal requirements, and state certification procedures.

Evacuation

Help people learn to exit homes, offices, and other buildings regularly accessed, using both **primary and alternate ways out.** This is an ongoing process, since over time we all forget. Everyone also should be familiar with the alarm system, pull-stations, and maintaining smoke detectors.

When investigating fires, **never just open a closed door.** Check for smoke coming from around the door. Then, feel the doorknob and the top of the door for heat. If there is no evidence of fire, open the door slowly. If the door opens toward you, brace your shoulder against the door to counter possible pressure.

During an evacuation, **crawl low if there is any smoke.** Be familiar with the setting's emergency plan. Have a designated place outside the building to meet during evacuations.

fire drills

Training

Support people to practice fire drills regularly. Everyone's teamwork is important, as is mutual respect. Use the following sequence of drills to teach evacuation:
1. Walkthrough: to learn the procedures
2. Announced drill: to practice the procedure
3. Surprise drill: to evaluate the practice

use of a fire extinguisher

Fire Suppression

Portable fire extinguishers are an important line of defense against fire and should be readily available. **Do you and the people you support know right now where extinguishers are in the places you live and work?** They should be used only after everyone has safely escaped and the fire department has been called, and if the fire is small.

Different kinds of fires require different kinds of extinguishers. Be familiar with the extinguishers available. Combustible fires take water extinguishers called Type A; flammable liquid fires take Type B; electrical fires require Type C.

Most fire extinguishers work this way:
1. Pull the pin.
2. Aim the nozzle at the base of the fire.
3. Squeeze the handle.
4. Sweep from side to side.

People should practice with extinguishers where they work and live, and check each for variations on instructions. Be sure that extinguishers also are checked regularly for proper pressure.

Managing Stress

For all of us, the accumulation of day-to-day problems or the event of a major loss or crisis can cause considerable feelings of stress. Stress is a very individual reaction and varies with each of us. It is determined by the meaning we attach to what happens to us. Our body reacts physically to these perceptions.

All stress isn't bad. It even can help performance. Too much stress, though, hinders performance and can greatly restrict effectiveness and enjoyment of life.

People with disabilities can experience the same type of stress reactions that anyone does. It is important to understand stress and how to manage it—both for yourself in your role, and for the people with disabilities you support.

There are at least three types of approaches to managing stress. One is to maintain the good health practices discussed earlier such as **exercise and healthy eating.** Another is to **learn how to relax** both the body and the mind. A third way is to **work on changing the perceptions you develop about your situations.**

For example:

- Learn to distinguish what you can change and what is beyond your control.
- Think positively about situations and recognize that stress is temporary.
- Work together on solutions and alternative ideas, rather than blaming others.
- Don't expect perfection. Be realistic.
- Seek help from friends, relatives, professionals, or support groups when you need it.
- Exercise, eat right, and don't overindulge in alcohol, drugs, caffeine, or nicotine.
- Learn relaxation techniques such as stretching, meditation, or deep breathing.

> Managing stress involves healthy living, learning to relax, and perceiving situations as positively and realistically as possible.

Summary

Like all of us, individuals with disabilities need to maintain good health and safety practices to support their ability to experience personal wellness and fulfillment in life. It is also crucial to their success in working, living, and recreating in the community. Good hygiene, nutrition, and exercise, for example, relate strongly to a person's sense of well-being, health, and personal presentation. This in turn influences people's ability to make friends, find and keep jobs, contribute to their communities, and generally experience the richness of life.

In your role of enhancing the quality of life for people, you will need to understand and support good medical and dental care. You also will need to be competent in fire safety and stress management.

Anatomy Is Not Destiny

Partially as a result of my participation in the disability rights movement, I have come to better terms with my physical self...

My idea of physical well-being is simply living up to one's physical potential, and I hope to live up to mine. I have taken yoga, and I now have an exercise program supervised by a physical therapist whose approach is holistic. My increase in physical self-esteem has had side effects ... Now I buy many of my clothes in dress shops and only in my correct size ...the fact remains that I am an independent adult woman, which is one of the things I always wanted to be.

– Lisa Blumberg
The Boston Globe Magazine

Everyday Health and Safety

POSTSESSION REVIEW

Name _____   Agency _____
Program _____   Trainer_____
Date _____   Score _____

1. Why is cleanliness important to everyday health?

2. Name at least three food groups.

3. Many people have inactive lifestyles. Yet along with good hygiene and nutrition, regular _____ is important for physical and emotional health.

4. Briefly list and describe the three types of seizures.

5. During a seizure you should try to protect the person from getting hurt. True or False. What should be considered in making this decision?

6. What are three things you could do if you felt you or a person with whom you work was under too much stress?

7. List three steps you can take in preventing fires.

8. What are the steps for using most fire extinguishers?

9. During a fire evacuation you should:
   a. try to fight the fire
   b. try to get everyone dressed
   c. head for the nearest exit while staying close to the floor
   d. try to find the fire

10. Name three good personal dental care practices that are important for everyone.

Part F

Support Through Personal Empowerment

This orientation manual was designed to provide you with an **introduction** to your new role in services for people with disabilities. As pointed out, ideas about what this role should be have evolved dramatically with our greater sensitivity to individuality, a respect for the contributions of all people, community life, and normalization.

In some ways, this new conception of the direct service person has created questions within the service system in which you work.

- How successful are we in making residences real homes?
- How much time should people with disabilities spend in our "training" programs?
- How do we balance skill acquisition with community participation?
- How are we accountable to funders, families, and the people with disabilities we support, particularly with something such as promoting social relationships and quality of life?

> The evolution of disability services requires those of us who help people to be more facilitators of community supports than caretakers in place of those supports.

Enhancing Lives

As we try to answer these questions and clarify our role, we find ourselves viewing a direct service person as more of a life enhancer or facilitator. The idea of life enhancement is a large step beyond helping to take care of someone. It means **becoming aware** of the local community, its people, and its resources. It means **helping to access** those resources. It means **advocacy** when needed. It means **building bridges** to people, groups, and associations. And it means **creating networks** around and with a person with a disability so the individual participates as a citizen, neighbor, co-worker, and friend with something to contribute.

Family Support

One key part of that network is the family of the person with a disability. When a family member has a disability, most parents encounter many kinds of professionals, such as physicians, teachers, and case managers. Similarly, service workers meet many kinds of parents with varying needs and expectations. This can be challenging for a staff person. But it is a safe assumption that **the quality of support a person will receive rests on your ability to work well with his or her family.**

> An important role for disability professionals is to respect and support families and their decisions about their life, roles, resources, and future.

Family members are the ones who, next to the person with a disability her or himself, know the individual the best. We need to respect and use that knowledge. As service workers, we should be able to give insights and information to the family. Many families feel that their best support is a person who can help the family to:

- think of their family member with a disability as a person with dreams, hopes, and skills
- understand the person's strengths, aptitudes, and competencies
- view family networks as a source of support in community life
- come to respect the person's life goals and achievements

You can best achieve this by being someone who:

- listens and understands
- becomes involved with the whole family
- knows and informs the family about resources
- develops an overall view of family and individual needs
- helps coordinate services

All People Have Rights

Over the years, persons with disabilities have been vulnerable to mistreatment, exploitation, abuse, and neglect. They have been subject to experimentation and inhumane treatment in the name of science and education. Although the US Constitution protects the individual rights of all citizens, individuals with disabilities have needed increased protection under the law.

In order to define more specific rights, federal and state laws, as well as policies and regulations of state agencies, have been developed. These include federal anti-discriminatory laws such as the Americans with Disabilities Act, and state-defined rights and policies on access to appropriate services. In addition, federal and state court decisions have interpreted and further refined these acts. Rights may be thought of in two ways: as affirmative rights or protection from mistreatment.

Affirmative Rights

Affirmative rights detail areas of opportunities along with the supports needed to enjoy a decent quality of life. For example, all qualified and eligible persons with disabilities have the right to **effective and appropriate services.** These should be voluntary, not restrictive, and as close as possible to home.

Services also must be designed to meet individual needs and promote independence. For example, residential services should be in home settings with privacy, good nutrition, and access to daily recreational opportunities. People should be able to receive assistance as needed in daily living, communicating with others, and accessing community places.

A person or his or her legal guardian has the right to active participation in meetings to plan for the future and to make the ultimate decisions about services the person will receive. In any termination from services, there must be sufficient notice to the individual. The person must be informed as to why, and be able to challenge the decision.

People have the right to manage their affairs. For instance, an adult will decide on his or her own how to spend money and free time, and how to maintain and use personal possessions. An adult also may decide where and with whom to live or work, how to worship, and whether to vote.

Protection from Mistreatment

Whenever we support individuals, we also must take care to ensure they are not vulnerable to mistreatment. For example, persons with disabilities must be free from any act, either of negligence or intention, that exposes them to serious risk of harm. This includes interactions based on corporal punishment, physical or sexual abuse, or mental or verbal abuse leading to physical or emotional harm.

> **People with disabilities may need safeguards to ensure they realize their basic affirmative rights to the lifestyle of their choice.**

If it becomes essential to protect a person from harm, a court may intervene to limit some kinds of choices involved in affirmative rights, such as those related to certain medical treatment decisions. A guardian may be appointed to make other kinds of decisions in the best interests of the person as determined by a court. A payee of funds also may be established by the Social Security Administration if a person is determined to be unable to manage income from benefits.

Further rights within services and the regulations around reporting violations of rights are detailed in state policies, and a new staff

People with disabilities can be vulnerable to mistreatment or neglect, even by well-intentioned services, unless their human rights are actively safeguarded.

person must review and become familiar with them. Each agency providing services should have a clearly defined rights protection system.

In summary, persons with disabilities have the right to the **same quality of life in their community we all have**. Since they may need certain assistance to realize this, specific rights are spelled out to affirm opportunities and prevent exploitation, mistreatment, or neglect. If you have reason to believe that mistreatment has occurred, you are **obligated to report it.** You should review with your trainer the reporting requirements and procedures within your particular agency.

You also have an additional responsibility related to affirmative rights. You should assist individuals to make effective decisions about their lives by presenting options and information in ways each person can understand. You also should educate each individual about the likely consequences of choices made. But once someone has made an educated decision about his or her life, that decision should be respected, even if you might have chosen otherwise.

staff obligations to rights protection

Self-Advocacy and Empowerment

As we have learned, the services we provide should be based on the interests, needs, and preferences of the person with a disability and those who are close to him or her. The terms *empowerment* and *self-determination* have been used to represent this posture. But just what are the implications of true empowerment?

Some people view empowerment as the individual making choices about his or her life. Others state that the person must have the ability to control and direct funding and other resources. Still others point to the need to be informed, make decisions, and be able to change one's mind about a job or a living situation.

It is possible to exercise this type of control, but it is not easy given the structure of most service systems. Also, in many places, the resources available for support generally are limited and somewhat restricted in use by regulations. Finally, people with disabilities can still be subject to discrimination or, in some cases, simply be ignored.

These obstacles to empowerment have led to the development of *self-advocacy* (see A-14). Self-advocacy has been defined variously by organizations of self-advocates as "the act of speaking for oneself," as well as "working together for justice by helping each other take charge of (our) lives and fight discrimination."

One of the most effective ways to bring about change is to

self-advocacy

organize a grass roots coalition of people who are directly affected by the issue. For people with disabilities, learning to speak out about their desires and rights, and to point out mistreatment or neglect, can be the most important survival skill to learn.

As a service provider, you should take the position that each individual with whom you work should direct the service system. You then should act to ensure that this will occur whenever possible:

- Help the person and his or her family and friends to recognize and understand pertinent information of life preferences, job and home options, recreation, life skills, and other areas related to the person's desired lifestyle.

> "...I still have to beg and struggle to get chances to learn ... It's even worse for people who aren't as persistent as I am. They don't get anything at all ... We can learn. We can get jobs and support ourselves instead of being supported by taxpayers ..."
> – Roberta Gallant, People First of NH

- Work to build a relationship so that communication of informed choice from the person becomes easy and natural.
- Develop life experiences related to interests and skills in a variety of community settings for the person to directly experience.
- Represent the person in negotiations with others to realize the person's expressed wishes.
- Help the person to implement decisions around supports, services, and the use of financial resources.
- Help to arrange expressed preferences by the person for particular service providers, job coaches, residential staff, case managers, or others.
- Help to arrange expressed preferences by a person for a home, neighborhood, roommate, or home modifications.
- Help to arrange expressed preferences by a supported employee for particular job tasks, co-worker supports, or other job accommodations.
- Discover the learning style most effective for the person and explain it to those who will provide training and assistance.
- Maintain ongoing communication to stay informed of changing needs for support.
- Advocate for the continued career advancement for a supported employee within the business setting.
- Provide timely assistance when the person feels a need for a change.
- Listen and respond to the person's evaluation of his or her life and service supports.

To conclude, then, let's think of all that we have covered in this introductory manual. We have discussed developmental and other disabilities, and the philosophy and implementation of normalization. We have reviewed your role and the skills that will make you effective for teaching new behaviors and skills. And we have looked at good health and safety practices. There are many more topics to learn and much more in-depth information to study. You should develop an individualized plan for your own further growth and development with your supervisor or trainer.

On the following page is a summary of some important guiding principles found throughout this manual to use in making day-to-day decisions in your work.

Guiding Principles in Supporting Persons with Disabilities

- Strive to build and support personal relationships.
- Utilize natural supports as much as possible.
- Assist with community involvement of the person's choice.
- Support active participation, even if partial participation is necessary.
- Use non-intrusive, natural interventions, and avoid artificiality.
- Be sensitive to individual rights, particularly privacy, personal decision-making, and personal space.
- Help to maintain natural routines and rhythms.
- Be conscious of age appropriateness.
- Provide and educate about real choices and respect decisions made.
- Help people to experience life fully.
- Be active in respectful partnership with families.
- Maintain good health, safety, and medical practices.
- Utilize the power of modeling in your own behavior and self-presentation.
- Help the person learn functional skills by utilizing sound teaching methods.
- Be conscious of subtle images, postures, and language that can devalue people.
- Promote status, competencies, and personal growth.
- Work in the broad sense as an enhancer of quality in each person's life.

You have one of the most important positions and opportunities there is—enhancing the quality of life of another individual. Take the time to learn the tools and resources that will enable you to do the best job you can.

To share your comments and suggestions about this manual, please forward them to:
Dale DiLeo
Training Resource Network, Inc., PO Box 439, St. Augustine, FL 32085-0439
Telephone: 904-824-7121; Fax: 904-823-3554; E-Mail: info@trninc.com
Web-Site: www.trninc.com

© 2000 TRN, *Enhancing the Lives of Adults with Disabilities*

References

Blumberg, L. (1988). Anatomy Is Not Destiny. In *The Boston Globe Magazine*. January 3.

Browder, D. (1987). *Assessment of Individuals with Severe Handicaps*. Baltimore: Brookes Publishing Co., Inc.

Cassidy, K. (1992). *Fire Safety and Loss Prevention*. Los Angeles: Butterworth-Heinemann.

Gardner, J. and Chapman, M. (1985). *Staff Development in Mental Retardation Services: A Practical Handbook*. Baltimore: Brookes Publishing Co., Inc.

Gaventa, W., Ed. (1998). *Dimensions of Faith and Congregational Ministries with Persons with Developmental Disabilities and Their Families*. Princetown, NJ: Religion Division, American Association on Mental Retardation.

Gold, M. (1980). *Try Another Way*. Champaign, IL: Research Press.

Hagner, D. and DiLeo, D. (1993). *Working Together: Workplace Culture, Supported Employment, and Persons with Disabilities*. Cambridge, MA: Brookline Books.

Handal, K., M.D., Handal, K.A., and Dole, E.H. (1992). *The American Red Cross First Aid and Safety Handbook*. Boston: Little, Brown, and Company.

Hastings, J.A. (1999). *Voices in the Storm: A Personal Journey of Recovery from Mental Illness*. St. Augustine, FL: Training Resource Network, Inc.

Karpinski, M. (1988). *The Home Care Companion. Vol. 3: Creating Healthy Home Care Conditions: Infection Control*. Videotape. Medford, OR: Healing Arts Communications.

Kushner, H.S. (1988). *When All You've Ever Wanted Isn't Enough*. New York: Summit.

Langton, D. (1988). Part of the EMS Team. *Granite State Employment News*. June.

Larson, D., Ed. (1992). Mayo Clinic Family Health Book: *The Ultimate Illustrated Home Medical Reference*. New York: William Morrow.

Lovett, H. (1985). *Cognitive Counseling and Persons with Special Needs*. New York: Praeger Publishers.

McKnight, J. (1995). *The Careless Society: Community and Its Counterfeits*. New York: Basic Books.

Minnesota Governor's Council on Developmental Disabilities (1987). *A New Way of Thinking*. St. Paul, MN.

Minnesota Governor's Council on Developmental Disabilities (2000). *Parallels in Time*. St. Paul, MN.

Minnesota Governor's Council on Developmental Disabilities (1998). *Read My Lips: It's My Choice*. St. Paul, MN.

New Hampshire Developmental Disabilities Council (1989). *Pathways*. Concord, NH.

O'Brien, J. (1980). The Principle of Normalization: A Foundation for Effective Services. In Gardener, J.F., Long, L., Nichols, R., and Iagulli, D. (Eds.), *Program Issues in Developmental Disabilities*. Baltimore: Brookes Publishing Co., Inc.

Perske, R. and Perske, M. (1988). *Circles of Friends*. Nashville: Abingdon Press.

Perske, R. and Perske, M. (1980). *New Life in the Neighborhood*. Nashville: Abingdon Press.

The National Fire Protection Association, (1999). *Fire Safety for People with Disabilities*, Quincy, MA.

Schwartz, D. (1992). *Crossing the River: Creating a Conceptual Revolution in Community and Disability*. Cambridge: Brookline Books.

Summers, J.A. (1986). *The Right to Grow Up*. Baltimore: Brookes Publishing Co., Inc.

Wolfensberger, W. (1972). *Normalization in Human Services*. Toronto: National Institute on Mental Retardation.

Wolfensberger, W. (1983). *Social Role Valorization: A Proposed New Term for the Principle of Normalization*. Mental Retardation, 21, 234-239.

Worth, P. (1989). The Importance of Speaking for Yourself. In *The Association for Persons with Severe Handicaps Newsletter*, Vol. 15, 5, May, 1989.

Index